Stanley P. Maximovich, M.D., F.A.C.S. was in private practice in Plastic, Cosmetic, Laser and Reconstructive Surgery in the western suburbs (Hinsdale and Naperville) of Chicago.

Dr. Maximovich graduated with Honors from Brown University. While attending this Ivy League college, Dr. Maximovich played on the Ivy Football Championship Team of 1976. Dr. Maximovich has been inducted into the Brown University Athletic Hall of Fame with the 1976 Championship Team. He earned his M.D. from Rush Medical College in Chicago and served his general surgery and plastic surgery fellowship at Loyola University Medical Center in the western suburbs of Chicago.

Dr. Maximovich is an excellent speaker and has appeared in newspapers, on the radio and television. He has had numerous articles in the prestigious journal Plastic and Reconstructive Surgery, the premier international journal in plastic surgery. He is listed in "Guide to America's Top Plastic Surgeons" by Consumers' Research Council of America. Dr. Maximovich, also, has been honored with the Frederick Milton Thrasher Award.

With unique insight gained from his educational background, professional training, extracurricular interests and practical experience, Dr. Maximovich is delighted to share his advice on his 3rd Edition of "101 Ways To Feel and Look Great!: A Plastic Surgeon's Guide To Improve Your Life From The Inside Out".

Biddle House Publishing

*****

TESTIMONIALS

"In this fast paced world we tend to loose sight of everyday activities that add satisfaction to our lives. Dr. Maximovich has focused on this, as well as pride in ones appearance, as a way to boost well being. While reading this book we find that many aspects of our daily routine will provide overall fulfillment. This simple, yet insightful, approach to life allows us to realize that health and happiness are easily attainable." - Howard Heppe, M.D., Plastic Surgeon, Diplomate of the American Board of Plastic Surgery

"Dr. Stanley Maximovich's book, "101 Ways to Feel and Look Great" lays out easy-to-follow guidelines to improve your life. These useful methods don't cost a single penny; the only requirement is to make smarter decisions. I've been energetic and happy as a result and recommend this book to anyone who wishes to better their lives."- Patient

"Dr. Maximovich's book is a simple and fast read with advice that makes sense and is easy to follow." – Patient

*****

Biddle House Publishing

Library of Congress Catalog Card Number 2016910816

Maximovich, Stanley P, 1957-
101 Ways to Feel and Look Great!-3rd Edition by Stanley P Maximovich, M.D.,F.A.C.S.

ISBN 978-0-9671054-3-7

THIRD EDITION

*****

I dedicate this book to my wife, Kim; my son, Stan; my daughter, Lauren; my mother, Sophia; my father, who has passed away; my sisters', Janice and Sandy; and to the rest of my family.

*****

Warning And Disclaimer

This book has been produced to provide you with a wealth of information. Use it wisely and in good judgment. Seek the guidance of your family doctor, medical specialist or surgical specialist as needed before you partake in any new activity, diet or treatment. If other types of professionals need to be consulted before you go in any new direction in your life, do so. This book has been written to inform and educate. It contains information available only up to the printing date. The author and the publishing entity shall not be liable or responsible to any person or entity with respect to any loss or damages caused, or alleged to be caused, directly or indirectly by the information contained in this book.

*****

Contents

40. Read Other Books On Self Help
41. Surround Yourself With Beautiful And Elegant Things
42. Reach For The Heavens
43. Get Into A Groove
44. Never Stop The Learning Process
45. Take A Relaxing Shower
46. Enjoy The Moment At Hand
47. Learn To Get Yourself Motivated
48. Learn To Be Patient
49. Bring Your Manners With You Everywhere You Go
50. Learn How To Gain The Emotional Benefits Of A Vacation Without Actually Going On One
51. Try Not To Push The Panic Button
52. Endure The Rough Times Because You Will Get Through Them
53. Seek Out Athletic Competition
54. Concentrate On What You Can Do, Not On What You Cannot Do
55. Watch A Sporting Event And Act Like A True Fan Of The Game
56. Drink Plenty Of Fluid Each Day
57. If You Drink Alcohol, Drink Responsibly And In Moderation
58. Say No To Drugs
59. Take A Multivitamin And Mineral Supplement
60. Minimize Your Exposure To Catching A Cold And The Flu
61. Protect Your Skin From The Sun
62. Think Of Wearing Suntan Lotion Before You Go Out In The Sun Like You Think Of Wearing A Seat Belt Before You Drive In A Car
63. Who Should Protect Their Skin From The Sun? Children, Adults And Grandparents!
64. Do A Self Skin Exam Every Month
65. Have Abnormal Skin Growths Removed
66. Maximize The Condition Of Your Complexion
67. Treating Your Skin Well Now Will Have A Direct Impact On How It Will Look Years From Now
68. Working Out In The Outdoors Without The Proper Skin Protection Will Harm Your Skin In The Long Term
69. Stop Worrying About Not Getting A Dark Suntan
70. What About The More Exotic Ways To Smooth Skin?
71. Body Massage
72. What You See In The Mirror And Want Improved May Be Helped With Plastic Surgery
73. Fine Wrinkles And Blotchiness Of The Face Can Be Improved With Laser Skin Resurfacing
74. Laser Skin Resurfacing Can Be Repeated In The Future
75. Chemical Peels Can Also Be Used To Treat Fine Wrinkles And Blotchiness Of The Facial Skin
76. Renova Cream
77. Eyelid Puffiness and Bagginess Can Be Improved To Create A More Youthful Appearance
78. Facial Skin Sagging Can Be Improved With A Face-Lift
79. Neck Sagging And Fat Excess Can Be Improved Through A Combination Of Skin Tightening, Muscle Tightening And Liposuction
80. The Effects Of Aging On The Forehead Skin Can Be Improved
81. Wrinkling Of The Skin Between The Eyes Can Be Improved With Botox, Muscle

Removal Or Laser Skin Resurfacing
82. Thin Lips Can Be Made Fuller, Thick Lips Can Be Made Thinner
83. Noses Can Be Reshaped, Nasal Breathing Improved
84. Ears That Are Too Prominent Can Be Reshaped
85. Chins Can Be Made More Prominent
86. For Women, Breasts That Are Too Large Can Be Made Smaller And The Symptoms Related To Large Breasts Improved
87. For Women, Small Breasts Can Be Enlarged, Sagging Breasts Lifted
88. Breast Reconstruction Can Create A New Breast, Replacing What Has Been Lost Due To Cancer
89. For Men, Large Breasts Can Be Reduced
90. Sagging Upper Arms Can Be Tightened
91. Fat Excess Of The Abdomen Can Be Decreased With Liposuction
92. Excess Skin And Fat Rolls Of The Lower Abdomen Can Be Removed With A Tummy Tuck
93. Bulging Thighs Can Be Reduced With Liposuction
94. A Bulging Buttock And Fat Excess Around The Knees And Calves Can Be Improved With Liposuction
95. Have Any Spider Veins And Varicose Veins Of The Legs Treated
96. Shape The Eyebrow Hairs To Look As Attractive As Possible
97. Help Is Available For Facial Acne Scars And Chicken Pox Marks
98. Unwanted Tattoos Can Be Treated
99. What To Do About Nasty Scars
100. Spend Your Youth Attaining Wealth, Spend Your Wealth Attaining Youth
101. It Is Your Time To Feel And Look Great

*****

101 Ways To Feel And Look Great!

1.

Eat The Right Food, Follow A Proper Diet

You are what you eat. If you are primarily eating the wrong food, you may not like how you feel and look. By eating the right food and reasonable portions you will feel and look better immediately after your next meal and on into the future.

Why will you feel and look better on your very next meal? By eating a better meal and not overstuffing yourself, you'll lose that bloated feeling you usually have. You will not have to undo your belt and unbutton your pants to allow your stomach to stretch like you usually do. Try looking in the mirror to see how great you look next time you stuff yourself. Now use that mental image for motivation.

Eating the proper portions of well-balanced food puts you on the road to freedom. You will also suffer fewer episodes of indigestion. Decrease your total calorie intake. Did you know that laboratory mice fed a low-calorie diet outlive mice fed a high-calorie diet? Food that is high in fat or sugar content is not the best for you. Eat fruits and vegetables at least two to three times a day. Don't count deep-fried vegetables as a healthy cooked vegetable.

Start by making your very next meal a well-balanced meal and don't stuff yourself. A well-balanced meal should have proportionate amounts of foods from the five basic food groups.

The five basic food groups are 1) Fruits 2) Vegetables 3) Bread, rice, pasta or cereal 4) Cheese, yogurt or milk and 5) Fish, meat, chicken, turkey, or eggs. A sixth group; fats, oils and sweets, which should be used sparingly, has been added to the original five basic food groups.

Try a well-balanced diet for at least one week and don't over-eat. Think of how you'll feeling at the end of one week. You will notice you're feeling better for the first hour after each meal and throughout the rest of the day. Are you having fewer episodes of indigestion? Do you no longer have to undo your pants belt after eating? Have you stopped groaning after meals? When you step on the scale you may find that you have not only not gained weight, but that you've also lost some. You have just taken a giant step forward. Consult your doctor regarding your diet. He or she can give you further advice about your particular needs. By following your new diet and the other advice in this book, you will be on your way to feeling and looking great!

2.

Minimize Snacks

Why do you eat snacks? You may eat them when there is nothing to do, for the pure enjoyment of the taste, to reward yourself or just for the heck of it. Sometimes a snack will stare you right in the face when you walk past the pantry. Maybe you snack because there's still time before you ate your next meal or because you purchased a stack of candy from your neighbor's child who was going door-to-door for a fund-raiser. Perhaps you snack when you're feeling sorry for yourself or when your favorite sports team has won or lost. You may eat certain snacks because everyone else eats them or because you can't get the thought of eating them off your mind.

Regardless of your motivation, snacking may have become part of your daily routine. You might be eating snacks more that once a day and possibly in excess each time. Everyone has there own definition of snacking, but it means eating a light meal between regular meals. Snacks usually consist of chocolate, ice cream, chips, candy, or even leftovers from the refrigerator.

The point is to minimize snacks. They generally aren't the proper foods to be eating in the first place. If you are not eating healthy food for your regular meals, you only worsen things by eating unhealthy snacks. If you cannot eliminate the ritual of snacking then snack on boring (but healthy) things like carrots, bananas, apples, and other fruits.

You will feel and look better if you can accomplish this, so do it! Should you find yourself thinking "...but my snack tastes so good...," remember this story: Laboratory animals were allowed to consume as much cocaine as they wanted, anytime of the day or night. They all ended up consuming as much as possible because it makes them feel so good when they did it, but they all died an early death as a result.

3.

Get Exercise

Learn to exercise properly so you don't hurt yourself. Start and continue at a slow and steady pace and do not try to increase the intensity of your work out too soon. If you injure yourself by straining your back, neck, arms or legs you will usually stop exercising until you recover, which could take weeks or months. By then you may have lost your motivation to work out. All the time you lost while recovering could have been spent continuing your exercise program. Remember the story of the tortoise and the hare. The tortoise ultimately won the race because the slow, steady and continuous pace wins out over the long term.

Exercise, if done properly and in moderation, will allow you to gain a greater sense of well-being. You feel better about your body as it starts to look better in the mirror. You will find yourself clearing your mind of negative thoughts, especially during your workout. You will notice you have more energy. Ultimately you will live longer.

You don't need to set aside an hour or two each day to start an effective workout program. Start with only 5 minutes a day. That's right, only five minutes a day! Why? Because you want to avoid getting discouraged in the beginning. A common reason people stop exercising is that they hurt themselves within the first two weeks of their new exercise program. Their bodies were not in any shape to start exercising at full speed. Also, if a person spent too much time each day driving to and from the health club and then waiting to use the equipment, he or she may feel the whole process is too time consuming. Lack of time is no excuse for not working out. Start exercising in your bedroom and your workout will be finished before you could travel to the health club and even before all your other important daily commitments get in your way. You may be thinking, "But I want to start with a one-hour work out and build from there." Be patient. You will reach that level if you are so inclined, but get there by minimizing your chance of injury and strain. Do not get discouraged by trying too much too soon. Exercise should be a lifelong activity, so start slow and easy.

Look at it this way. You have to get in good shape simply to start any exercise program you are considering. Do not purchase or use any type of home exercise machine until you can use it without injuring yourself. First get fit before you start working out on your home weight machine, rowing machine or treadmill. Then build up your level of fitness before starting on some of the machines at the health club. Machines that force you to exercise multiple body parts simultaneously should be only used once you are in better shape to tolerate them. A prominent but out of shape heart surgeon wanted to get into better shape so he suggested that we work out together at a health club he had joined but never used. I told him exactly what I have just told you. He needed to first start on a simple five minute a day exercise program. He could build from there over a period of months. I warned him not to start with the type of exercise program he envisioned starting because it would be too much too soon.

Depending on your age and state of health, you may need to consult with your physician before starting any exercise program. Your physician can decide which of the following exercises you should exclude and what additional exercises you should include. Start out with five minutes of exercise three days a week. Build up by five minutes every other week to a time commitment you can consistently manage. If you are so inclined, you can work out up to five days a week but rest is very important. Start with five sit-ups, five push-ups and five jumping jacks. This is considered a single set of exercises. On the third week try to do two sets of exercises. This means that after completing five sit-ups, five push-ups and five jumping jacks, you do another five sit-ups, five push-ups and five jumping jacks. You will then have done two sets of exercises.

Every other week you can increase the sets or the number of each exercise per set. Increase only to what you can tolerate. After a while you'll find yourself doing a total of twenty to thirty or more sit-ups, push-ups and jumping jacks each during your exercise session. Just remember: Do not start doing thirty sit-ups at one time if you haven't done that before. Start slow and easy and build up your strength.

Run in place for five seconds between each exercise. On the third week increase this to ten seconds between each exercise. Try fifteen seconds between each exercise by the fifth week. You can include any of your favorite exercises into this program, even outside running. After a month or two you'll find yourself ready to tackle the health club where, if you wish, you can enter a more serious exercise program under supervision. You can build up your physical fitness, because you now have a method of building your strength and endurance.

You will find that you will feel sore within the first several days or weeks following this program. The soreness is absolutely to be expected but by continuing the workouts you will find it eventually lessen. This workout is designed to minimize serious injuries, so there are no heavy weights to lift and strain yourself with. This exercise program will also build your strength and endurance for sports or social activities like tennis, golf and dancing.

If you simply want to take a daily walk for exercise, do it! Another option is to walk up a flight of stairs and down two flights instead of using the elevator at work. Imagine if you only did the minimum - five sit-ups, five push-ups, five jumping jacks and running in place for five seconds between each exercise - three days a week, but you did this consistently for one year. Think how you will feel and look in the mirror if you only did this compared to no activity!

4.

Stretch Out Before And
After A Workout

In Chapter 3 you learned a method of exercise that you can follow the rest of your life. Now it's important to add stretching out both before and after your exercise routine. Why? Because stretching out will help minimize your risk of muscle pulls, ligament strains and overall soreness and stiffness. It will allow you to continue your exercise program with a minimum of downtime.

In my high school athletic training I understood the importance of stretching out. At that time stretching out was something done only before the workout. But when I went into training for the 1976 football season at Brown University, our head trainer incorporated something totally new into our work-outs. At the end of each practice, he simply made us repeat the entire set of stretching exercises we had done at the beginning of the session.

Our trainer had learned the benefits of post-workout stretching months earlier during his trip to Japan with the USA Olympic team. He found that the athletes who also stretched out after practice suffered fewer injuries and tolerated the strenuous workout with less prolonged soreness and stiffness than athletes who did not follow this routine. To my amazement, by simply stretching out also after each practice session, I experienced less soreness and stiffness than I had in all my previous years of athletic training.

Incorporate stretching out both before and after you exercise. You may need to consult with your physician before getting started. Begin with neck rotations; rotate your head in a full circle five times going clockwise, then five times going counterclockwise. Next extend your arms out to the sides; rotate both arms in a full circle five times going in one direction and five times in the opposite direction. Continue with trunk rotations; rotate your upper body in a full circle while your legs remain stationary. Do the trunk rotations five times in a clockwise direction and five times counterclockwise. Follow these with side stretches; bend at the waist as far to the left as you can go down five times and then to the right side as far as you can go down five times.

Now on to the toe touches. Stand straight up with your hands on your hips, and then bend at the waist while trying to touch your toes. At the beginning, you may not be limber enough to bend over all the way, so be careful not to strain yourself. Start by doing these five times. After each toe touch, reach up to the sky with both hands and stand on your tiptoes, then bring your hands onto your hips. Repeat this five times.

You can include any of your own personal stretching exercises into this routine. Start by doing each stretching exercise a minimum of five times and build up repetitions as you do the rest of the exercises. You'll soon notice an improvement in your level of flexibility.

5.

Stop Smoking

The easiest decision to make, but one of the hardest things to do, is to quit smoking. If you currently don't smoke but have been thinking about starting, don't do it! Smoking can lead to many major health problems, including heart disease, lung disease and cancer. It will make your complexion look more harsh and aged and will stain your teeth. Your breath, clothes, car, home and office will have an unpleasant odor of smoke. If you smoke, you will become more easily fatigued, making it more difficult for you to exercise properly. Smoking will simply not allow you to feel and look your best.

Even if you have been smoking for years, you can actually reverse the non-cancerous damage to your lungs by no longer smoking. By stopping smoking, it will improve the condition of your lungs. Although it may take your body up to ten years to reverse the lung damage caused by smoking, it can happen.

Smoking will make your skin look much older because direct contact with cigarette smoke damages your facial skin. Have you ever looked at the ceiling of a house or an office where people smoke? You'll see that the ceiling is yellowed and discolored. If the ceiling looks like that from cigarette smoke, just imagine what it can do to your skin! Facial skin is also affected by cigarettes because the smoke inhaled contains substances that enter your circulatory system and decrease the blood flow to your skin. Decreased circulation to your facial skin will not allow your complexion to look as good as it should. If you have seen people with poor circulation to their lower legs, you know that the leg skin can look terrible as a result of decreased blood flow.

When I perform an operation on someone who smokes, I tell them that to have the best chance of healing, they have to stop smoking weeks before the procedure and must continue to not smoke for weeks afterward. If they are looking for an excuse to stop smoking then their upcoming procedure is a perfect reason.

Stop smoking and you'll soon notice the benefits. I didn't say it would be easy, but be faithful to yourself and it will occur. Imagine yourself if you stopped smoking today and then looked at yourself five and ten years from now. Imagine how much better you would feel and look than if you continued to smoke.

6.

Get Regular Checkups From Your Doctor

You have a direct influence over your health. Treat your body well. It is still important to have regular checkups with your doctor. There are important matters concerning your health which may only be identified or recognized by a physician with the aid of laboratory or other testing. Based on your personal and family medical history, your doctor will be able to determine the extent of the physical exam you need and order blood testing or other testing when necessary.

It's important to seek out a doctor's expertise with the goal of staying healthy and preventing problems from occurring or worsening. To maintain your health you have to count on yourself but also seek help from your doctor. Certain health problems which go unchecked may only get worse and lead to more serious conditions.

You may need to schedule a regular checkup with your doctor multiple times a year, once a year or less frequently. How often you need to have checkups will be determined and explained by your doctor who will consider such factors as your age, sex, personal and family medical history, physical exam findings and such. If you're due for your regular checkup, get on the phone and make that appointment. It's important if you want to make yourself feel and look your best!

7.

Minimize Boredom

Create a more interesting life for yourself. Was your life less boring years ago? Where you involved in more activities back then? Did you have more zip in your step and more pride in your stride? Did you feel you accomplished more in the past but now seem to accomplish less? Does it seem like everyone else is doing the fun things in life but you're not? Do you feel like you wouldn't like to hang around with yourself if given the opportunity?

You need to reassess how the simple things in your life have made you happy, kept you busy and minimized your boredom. Remember when you were in the third grade and you could play for hours with a simple toy? You used your imagination and created hours of fun for yourself. If you had a friend over, it was even better because you both could get into the game of make-believe. It was all part of having fun.

When was the last time you felt like you were using your imagination and creativity? Are you now locked in a rigid lifestyle which doesn't allow you to be imaginative? If the answer is "yes," you may now know why you can't shake that feeling of boredom. Are you bored by the same activities that other people find exciting? If the answer is "yes," you need to think about just having fun on a more simplistic level.

Why does your dog jump with excitement when you take your dog on a simple car ride to the store? Your dog acts like it just won the lottery. You, on the other hand, feel like the car ride is just only another chore. You may have lost touch with simple pleasures in your life that can help minimize boredom. You may not have to change anything you're now doing in order to minimize your boredom. You may only have to change your attitude about what you're doing.

However, if you do need to increase your activities, then do it. Try building a model or collecting leaves and pressing them into a book. Try doing the very things that made you so happy when you were young. Tap into your imaginative and creative self. Both your attitude adjustment and bringing your creative side to the front will go a long way toward making you feel and look your best!

8.

Minimize Your Risk Of Having An Accident

Safety first. Accidents are the leading cause of death in the younger age groups. When you turn on the evening news, how many times do you hear of people dying or getting injured due to an accident? You need to recognize where accidents are likely to occur during your daily activities and take steps to minimize your risks. You obviously have no control over some accidents but many are preventable. If you really understood before an accident all the pain and suffering you'd experience, you'd do everything possible to prevent that accident from happening in the first place.

Princess Diana of England died in a car accident in France. She was not wearing her seat belt. Only one person out of the four in her car was wearing a seat belt. That one person survived and was ultimately able to walk and talk. You can never be too cool or too rich to not wear a seat belt.

The state of Illinois requires that seat belts be worn but there is a poor compliance with this law. Even though people know that it's better to wear a seat belt, they still choose not to do so. The reason? They don't understand ahead of time all the pain and suffering they'll have to endure if they're in a car accident. If they understood, they'd wear a seat belt to prevent serious injury.

If you crashed into a wall at 60 miles per hour without a seat belt, you probably wouldn't expect to survive. Did you know that you can create the same level of impact if you're only going 30 miles per hour in your car and drive head on into another car traveling at 30 miles per hour? You add the two speeds together to get the total impact speed of 60 miles per hour, which is equivalent to hitting a wall all by yourself at 60 miles per hour.

You now know that even if you're not traveling fast, a head-on collision with another car can be the equivalent to a very high speed crash.

Early in my surgical training I was required to treat patients who had been in car accidents. It was common to see more than one person involved in each accident. As the stretchers were rolled into the emergency room, if the patients were conscious, not complaining and looked in good shape, I knew they probably had on their seat belts. Patients who, on quick inspection, were in much worse shape usually were not wearing seat belts.

The point? The extent and severity of the accident is huge if you're not wearing your seat belt. If you have passengers with you, don't pull out of the drive way unless everyone in the car has buckled up their seat belts. I am often reminded that there are some truly preventable accidents. This occurs every time I perform plastic surgery on a pretty girl's face to correct the damage sustained by going into a car's windshield. The girl typically was not wearing a seat belt. It does not make sense for you to do all the proper things to make yourself feel and look great yet every day put yourself at risk of serious injury in a car accident by not wearing a seat belt.

It's also incredible how many people burn themselves with hot water or on the flame of the stove while cooking, break their leg because they fell off the roof while working on a minor project, or fall off a ladder and suffer serious injury even though they were only a few feet above the ground. Minimize the pain, suffering and scars by prevention in your daily life.

9.

Get Your Financial House In Order

Your financial health can have a direct impact on how you feel and look. If you're always worrying about financial matters, this will weigh you down and prevent you from ever enjoying the moment in which you are now living. If you think that you'll start to relax some time in the future, realize that you may never live to reach that time. Regardless of the type of job or business you currently have or will have some day, there will always be the potential for financial concern. Financial health needs to be thought of as part of your general health. You must work to achieve and maintain good financial health just like you must work on your own good physical health. Plan to maximize your financial health.

Train yourself to work on your financial house on a regular basis. Reevaluate your finances once a week, once a month, as often as necessary to do the best job. Are you borrowing money with the lowest interest rate possible? Are you putting any money you have saved into areas which give you the highest interest rate but with the type of safety that makes you comfortable? You already know you should be doing this sort of self assessment.

Get control of your finances. Take the necessary time to regroup if you feel like you are not headed in the right financial direction. Once your path is redirected, give yourself some time to allow things to work out.

If you feel your personality, health and emotions are being dragged down by your financial situation, do something about it. Don't let it turn into a bottomless pit. Take action. Getting your financial house in order will help you clear negative thoughts out of your life and you'll feel like you have more control over yourself. You will feel better because an emotional heaviness will be relieved or at least lessened; and you'll notice that you are looking better in the mirror because you have shed your concerned look.

If your financial house is already in order congratulations! Keep it up! You still have to work on it on a regular basis to maintain it. Getting your finances in order will do wonders for the way you feel and look.

10.

Pay Attention To Your Loved Ones

Pay attention to your loved ones. You know who they are and that they are on your side. They want you to do your best and be successful. By taking the support they offer, you can gain a great deal of strength from them. Although they want you to win, they'll be waiting for you, win or lose. Spend more time talking to them and listening when they talk to you. Remember that they are there for you now and will always be there for you in the future.

Keep your loved ones near you instead of going the distance alone. In the long run, there is nothing to be gained by ignoring those who love you. Your growth as an individual is helped by what you learn from your relationships with others. But if you cannot pay more attention to those who are most important in your life, how can you pay attention to total strangers? If you are not treating your loved ones with respect, genuine interest and caring, how are you treating yourself and others outside your family? By being better to your loved ones, you will learn to be better toward yourself and the rest of humanity.

Amaze yourself with how much enjoyment you'll derive from talking to those you love. Get involved with your loved ones and you'll find out how little you actually know about what is currently going on in their lives. Listen when they talk to you. In today's world there is an overabundance of distracting information being shoved into your face all the time. For example, don't fall into a trap of watching too much TV. It may be distracting you from spending time with those who are important in your life. If you have the television on when you are trying to communicate with someone you love, will you listen primarily to the TV instead of your loved one? Open your lines of communication by reducing the obstacles.

People who love each other can share a great deal of emotional support. You and your loved ones should derive strength from each other. Everyone can use a shoulder to lean on in times of trouble. Pay attention to your loved ones because they are there for you for the rest of your life. They can give you strength, courage and endurance; and their love will go a long way toward making you feel and look your best.

11.

Stop Complaining

That's right. I said, "Stop complaining!" I'm not talking about the type of complaining that creates positive and constructive change. That's constructive criticism. I'm talking about the type of complaining that's only negative, not constructive. It is selfish in nature and can lead to hurt feelings. When you complain, you're responsible for the negative environment in which you must then exist in. You stop growing and maturing as an individual. Complaining about your own life does not lead to a resolution. If you're a constant complainer, other people want to run away as soon as they see you coming.

You must learn and practice constructive criticism if you want to stop complaining. If you see the need for improvement or change in something around you, whether it's for others or yourself, don't complain about it. Learn to provide constructive criticism. Explain why you feel there is a need for change and state what your suggestions are to create such a change. If the constructive criticism regards someone else and you are asking them to change be understanding. You may initially get a lot of resistance. Of course, if your constructive criticism involves yourself, you may also initially be resistant to following your own advice. Don't just complain about your life. Provide yourself with constructive criticism and act on the changes that need to be accomplished.

Complaining is not positive. It may be used in a destructive way only to hurt someone. There is no point in complaining simply to create ill will. Have you ever watched someone who was only complaining and not providing constructive criticism? Did you feel that the person was looking or feeling his or her best? While people are complaining, they appear unattractive, unappealing, unsociable, unhealthy and generally undesirable. They leave an unpleasant taste on your emotional taste buds.

Do you find that your complaining is stopping you from growing and maturing as an individual? Does it get in the way when you try to communicate with someone? If these things are true, remember that you have control over your complaining. You can change, so do it.

Stop complaining. Teach constructive criticism to people who are complainers. Revise the way you look at things, other people and yourself. Be constructive from now on in your thoughts and comments to others as well as yourself. The less you complain, the more attractive, appealing, social and generally good-natured you will become. Stopping yourself from complaining will lead you toward feeling and looking great.

12.

Use Action Over Indecision

Action over indecision will lead to results. In all the topics I have discussed and the ones to follow, if no action is taken, you'll receive no benefits. Being passive does not lead to self improvement. You, personally, must get the ball rolling. You can keep delaying your decision on making yourself feel and look great but there is no reason to do so. Stop wasting time trying to talk yourself out of doing something good for yourself. You could have already gained the benefit by taking action.

If you take no action, you cannot expect the results you desire. If you have been thinking about minimizing your snacking but have not actually done it, you have experienced no real benefit. You must take action by truly cutting back on the snacks because only then are you helping yourself. Take the necessary steps to accomplish your goals.

Do you have goals that you never really try to achieve? If so, don't consider them goals but rather call them your fantasies. A fantasy is something you create out of your imagination, something that you usually will never see in your life. A goal, however, is something you define before you even get started achieving it. Once you have a goal in mind, you can focus on the actions which are necessary to achieve your goal.

You must get the ball rolling. Don't count on someone else to do it for you. Once you're inspired to take action, do the work that's necessary. Being inspired is only the first part. You must then put forth a serious effort. When people who don't want to improve themselves are given aid, the result is failure. A person has to begin with the desire to improve.

Stop being the driving force responsible for your life of indecision. Change this by defining your goals and taking action now. You will find taking action leads to a more productive life. Because it becomes less of a chore to do things you previously thought were too difficult to accomplish, you get more things done in a shorter period of time.

Taking action will soon become easier than being indecisive. You'll be more willing to put forth an effort when you can define your goals and the steps needed to reach them. Taking action will put you on your way to feeling and looking great.

13.

Get In Contact With Your Religious/Spiritual Self

If you're already in contact with your religious/spiritual self, keep it up. Strengthen it. If you've lost contact with this part of your life, work to get it back. If you never had it in the past, get it now. You need to live your life with a purpose. When you feel good about your inner self and your future, it will reflect on your outward appearance and how you feel physically.

Being in contact with your religious/spiritual self means being in contact with God and your soul. This is not something you only do one hour a week on Sunday morning. It is the way you conduct yourself, the way you live your life and the way you treat others.

You need purpose in your life to make it more fun, exciting and challenging. Each day will have more importance to you as the old days of only going through the motions vanish.

You'll follow a clearer and concise path. You'll be able to help others because you know how to help yourself. Lead by example. As you continue to learn to help yourself, you'll be able to pass this knowledge on to others.

By getting in contact with your religious/spiritual self, you will start to feel better about your inner self. You will also have better insight into others around you. All this will lead to a more radiant outward self.

14.

Stop Thinking You Are Unlucky

Have you analyzed yourself and decided that you've been unlucky in life? The truth is you are not really unlucky. Although you might feel that your lot in life it is not that great, there are others who may envy you. You may not realize it but others may be wishing they had what you currently have. It's difficult to rely on luck to get through your whole life. Excluding the big lottery and things of that nature, work and dedication - not luck - are what ultimately will lead you to your destination.

All people want to better themselves. Just don't rely on luck to do it for you. Your life may actually be pretty good right now but you just don't appreciate it. It often takes hardships to make you finally realize how good your life really is. Hardship is a normal part of life that you must assume will happen at some time. When it occurs, you must have strength, courage and endurance to get through it.

Do you get everything you work toward? The answer is no. Do people you see in the news, movies, or on television have everything they want? The answer is no. They may have incredible fame and fortune, well above what you have but they still may feel they have not gotten what they deserve. They may feel that they have been unlucky while you feel that they could not have been any luckier.

Though you may not reach your top goal all the time, think of how high you've climbed. Work and dedication are what is needed. If you don't want to work for your goals, understand you've made a choice. Your decision was not to take action. That's OK. You don't have to accomplish absolutely everything in your lifetime.

When other people do apply work and dedication and accomplish what you had once thought about doing, be happy for them. Don't feel you are unlucky and they're lucky. They made the decision to work toward something and did the necessary steps to achieve their goals. You can use this to your understanding that work, and not luck, is the answer.

You are not unlucky. In fact, many around you probably feel you're lucky for your place in life. But hardship will occur and you cannot avoid it. Dedicate yourself to what you want to accomplish. Don't rely on fate alone to get you there. If you dedicate yourself to working toward your goals, you will find yourself feeling and looking better.

15.

Put Positive Thoughts In Your Head

Every time you think of negative thoughts or actions get them out of your head. If you start to think too negatively, it will be of no benefit to you. Negative thoughts can lead to anxiety, stress and ill health. They usually don't accomplish anything productive. Negative thoughts only leave you worrying about bad things that might, or might not, happen.

If you let these negative thoughts stay in your head too long, you'll find yourself concentrating on them and applying your full attention to them. Once you are at this point, you usually will allow them to play out fully to some negative outcome. You might never have imagined you could spend so much time thinking negatively, but you can.

You can control negative thoughts. The next time one creeps into your mind simply don't think about it any further. Think instead about something that's pleasant, fun, exciting, enjoyable, or something that makes you feel good. You can fall back on the same pleasant thought every time a negative thought occurs. Even though you start thinking about something else, you'll still find that negative thought trying to pop back into your head. Keep working on pushing negative thoughts out of our mind.

You really have to work at keeping negative thoughts out. It takes effort and patience on your part to do it effectively. It may not work the first time you try. It may take time before you become good at it. But once you learn to suppress negative thoughts, keep it up. Your mind should be your greatest ally, not an enemy.

Keeping out negative and unproductive thoughts is not the same thing as creating a method of problem solving in your head. When you problem solve, you think about how to correct something. You think about the steps needed to accomplish something and about the possible scenarios that could result. Depending on the potential outcome, you may have to think through how to correct the resultant scenario. Problem solving involves a plan to resolve a negative situation. It is productive and leads to action and results. If a negative thought needs problem solving, then problem solve. Don't just allow the negative thought to overcome you. In and of themselves negative thoughts are not productive. They don't lead to action or positive results. Negative thoughts only lead to more negative thoughts.

Get the negative thoughts out of your head and replace them with positive thoughts. Another option is to get busy so you are not thinking about anything in particular. Learn to recognize the difference between an issue which needs problem solving versus a destructive negative thought. Problem solve an issue, then get on with your life. Push a bad thought out of your head and keep it out. The more you train yourself to do this, the better you'll get at it. Eliminating negative thoughts will go a long way toward making you feel and look great.

16.

Get Some Quiet Time

You need to give yourself quiet time, regardless how hectic your day. No matter how swamped with work you are, you need to have some peace and quiet. It is important to shut everything out around you for brief periods to recharge your emotional batteries. Quiet time doesn't need to be productive. In fact, in many cases it is most productive to try not be productive during your quiet time. It is good to simply step away from the action. Allowing time for being completely nonproductive, to not do anything in particular except let time slip away is good for you. It's one of the luxuries of having quiet time. If you are getting quiet time, enjoy it for what it is worth. It is a chance to relax.

Choose a good place to get quiet time. Don't park yourself in the kitchen where everyone in your family will be walking through asking you questions, asking you to do things, asking you for money, asking you what you are doing, or asking you why you aren't doing anything. This is the wrong place for quiet time. The place for quiet time should actually allow you to experience peace and quiet.

There is an art and a science to getting quiet time. You may have to be creative to establish a location where you get the most benefit out of your quiet time. Every opportunity during the day where there is a slowdown in what you are doing will lend itself to quiet time. When you are home, you'll find that certain rooms are better than others. Sometimes just sitting in front of a television by yourself, not paying attention to anything in particular, will do it.

Do not feel guilty about having quiet time. Don't feel guilty that so many important things will be passing you by while you're relaxing. Don't worry that you are being lazy because you care about yourself and want this quiet time just for you. Take advantage of it.

Most professional sports don't allow their athletes to compete year round. The seasons are too grueling to expect athletes to continue year after year with no downtime in between them. If they had no downtime to rest and recovery from their work, most athletes would be significantly limited in how long they could compete. Many would only be able to compete for only a few years and would not be able to make a career in sports. Think of yourself as one of these professional athletes. You cannot continue to grind away endlessly with no down time. If you want to be at your peak performance, you require the proper rest and quiet time.

It is important to not look tired, dragged out, frustrated and anxious. You shouldn't look frazzled all the time. If you're not rested and in the right frame of mind for the important events in your life, you will not do your best. Set aside quiet time for yourself. It will make you feel and look great.

17.

Take A Nap

Taking a nap when you feel like it is great. It gives you your needed down time and elevates your spirits. A nap provides a natural lift that energizes you for the rest of the day. You'll probably find yourself getting more things accomplished after your nap because you're no longer tired. An effective nap may be as short as fifteen minutes or up to several hours long. If you're feeling tired and barely keeping focused it may be more productive to first take a one hour nap followed by two hours of productive activity, rather than pushing yourself for three hours feeling tired and accomplish very little. Don't let only the very young benefit from taking a nap - do it yourself!

If you are only able to take a nap on the weekend, do it then. If you find that you're not feeling rested and better after a nap, you are napping incorrectly. You don't want to wake up with a sore neck or a headache because you're napping on a chair or couch that's not comfortable for sleeping. If taking a nap in your bed makes you feel your best, then switch to your bed for all your naps.

Getting that natural, energized lift from a nap is wonderful. You'll no longer need to drink huge quantities of caffeinated products to stimulate yourself. Taking an effective nap will reduce your dependence on caffeine and you won't need to consider taking an over-the-counter pill to pep you up and make you feel less sleepy during the day. If you need to take a fifteen minute nap at lunch time each day in your office, then do it. It's worth it if it makes you feel less sleepy in the afternoon and more productive. Stuffing yourself at the lunch table can also make you feel very tired several hours after you eat. You may need to eat smaller quantities of food at one time or fewer sugar-laden products to control this.

Why should only the young benefit from taking a nap? An adult should also benefit. Dogs always seem to have plenty of energy to run and play for hours. They never seem to tire out when you come home to play with them. The reason they have so much energy is that they get an incredible amount of rest all day long. While they wait for you to come home from work, all they do is lay around expending no energy.

There's nothing wrong with taking a nap during the day to boost your energy level, even though you feel you're getting enough sleep at night. If you're not getting enough sleep at night, then napping during the day may give you the rest you missed. First, however, it is important to determine why you are not sleeping at night and then try to correct that. You may need to seek out your physician's advice. Getting a good night's sleep is important to maintain your health.

Take a nap. You deserve it. You will be impressed how much better you'll start feeling. It will be like having released untapped energy and stamina. Look in the mirror and see the difference. A nap can go a long way toward making you feel and look your best.

18.

Put On Background Music

Put on background music whenever you have the opportunity. Whether you're at home, at work, in the car, on vacation or elsewhere, dial in a great radio station, play your IPOD or play a CD. If you can create your own music by playing the piano or another instrument, do it. Background music will make your day seem more effortless by lifting your mood, soothing your soul and make you feel good. Music can give you positive energy, especially if you hear a particular song that has a lot of meaning for you. Music is a strong emotional stimulant. It may remind you of a pleasant event that occurred at the same time you first listened to that specific song or artist. You can harvest some of your most pleasant memories from the music you listen to.

Fit the background music to your mood. If you're working on a project and want to feel calm, then play smooth jazz. If your mood is happy and stimulated, you may want fast, loud, upbeat music. If you're in a reflective mood, thinking about how much you enjoyed your junior and senior year in high school, you may want to play music from that period in your life. There is no single type of music that's perfect for all your different moods.

Putting on background music to make yourself feel better accomplishes great things. You're treating yourself to one of the truly wonderful experiences in lives. Music has, and always will have, a strong, positive impact on people. You must remember to listen to it in order to enjoy it.

If you're in a bad mood after work, you know the power of music. It can alter your mood during the drive home and make yourself feel better. To feel and look your best, make sure you incorporate music into the background of your live. Music acts in a constructive way on a conscious and unconscious level. It is there for your benefit. Take advantage of it!

19.

Get Your Relationships In Order

During the course of your life, you interact with many people. If you work, you have a certain relationship with the other people in your company. With your friends, you have a special relationship. With your family you have still another type of relationship. It is important to work toward having a good working relationship with all these people. You want to be positive when it comes to your relationships with others. To have success with different groups will lead to greater personal harmony. You'll find getting through your day more enjoyable. You'll be more appreciative of the opportunity to come in contact with others. As your relationships become more meaningful, you'll feel better about yourself.

If you're successful in your relationship with one group but are unsuccessful with another, improve this. If your relationships with your friends are great but your relationships with members of your family are not great, correct this. Try to understand why your family relationships may not be as good as they should be. Don't let years slip away without doing something about them. You can harbor unnecessary stress and anxiety because of bad relationships.

Take the initiative to get back into the good graces with whom you're having a difficult relationship. Don't say it's the responsibility of the other person to come to you and make things right again. You should be the one doing this. Learn to be the first to hold out the olive branch of peace. It will become much easier to improve your relationships with others if you are willing to do this. You'll be impressed that you can deal so effectively with people with whom you were previously in poor standing.

Improving your relationships with every person around you will actually make your day easier for many reasons. You will be more at ease and comfortable when you deal with these people. You'll find it more enjoyable to interact with others and they, in turn, will be more willing to help you. With more allies on your side offering you additional help, you might find yourself struggling less. You might find that all these people are actually fun to be around. You'll be enlightened by the fact that others can give you a great emotional lift that will make you feel great.

20.

Go To A Neighbor's House And Socialize

If you have free time today or tomorrow, drop by a neighbor's house and socialize. You don't have to plan this weeks in advance and write this in your calendar book. Simply stop over and ring the door bell. People make excuses that they no longer have time for such activity. This is nonsense. A neighborhood can feel unfriendly simply because no one takes the initiative to go over and start talking. You do not need to talk for hours. You can have an enjoyable conversation in minutes. In fact, some of the most memorable conversations you have all day may be during the few minutes spent with your neighbor. Unlike endlessly flipping through the television channels for hours, having no recollection what was said or what you watched, you will notice your conversation with another person has more impact on you. The few words that were spoken or ideas conveyed stay with you longer and can be very meaningful.

As a child, this is just what you'd do for hours a day, every day. In your childhood you called it playing. You'd hang out at your friend's house until it was time to go home and do homework, or eat or because it was getting too late. But as people grow up, they stop doing this and in doing so, they also stop doing something that used to give them great joy. The simple things that would bring them happiness as children are not continued into adulthood. People try to substitute more complex things for the simple things they've lost. Instead, stop and go back to these simple things and gain the benefits you've lost.

Making time in your day to socialize is important. You have to understand that this is one of the joys of being alive. As a human being, you have the ability to communicate with other people and gain from it. Don't turn your head away from your neighbor the next time you pass. Start a conversation. The more of an effort you make now, the easier it becomes later. If you need to make contact with your neighbors, don't think it will happen if you stay in your house. Get out of the house and take a walk. It's an easy opportunity to meet others and start up a conversation. The short time you are out and about socializing may become the most enjoyable part of your day.

Many people today realize that the feeling of community is lacking in their lives. There is a great push by developers of new communities to recreate that small town feeling. They want to recreate homes with front porches that are comfortable and big enough for you to actually want to sit there; build front sidewalks that are close enough to the houses for you to start a conversation with someone walking past while you're sitting on your front porch; and create an environment that encourages you to talk to others around you and makes you feel safe and comfortable.

Go back to that small town, small community, childhood feeling of what your neighborhood was once all about. This is what it should still be about. Make the effort to socialize with your neighbors. You will appreciate your neighborhood more and it will make you feel great.

21.

Reach A Comfortable Weight

If you currently feel you weigh too much or too little, you're probably thinking about changing your weight. You may have a goal of what you want your body weight to be but you have to be realistic about this change.

Is the problem too much weight? To do you the most good and help you maintain your new weight, a weight loss program should include ways to create a lifestyle change related to your eating habits. You'll probably lose your target amount of weight during the initial phase of your diet. The phase that takes inspiration on your part is to keep the weight off for the rest of your life. If, over time, you return to your old ways of eating, you'll gain back all the weight you initially lost.

Can you find a weight loss program which you can follow for the rest of your life? If so, do it and let everyone else know about it. This really would be considered a type of lifestyle program and not simply a weight loss program. A weight loss program helps you reach your desired weight but after that you must find a way to maintain your new weight.

You have to decide if you feel comfortable at your new weight. Do you feel good being at this reduced weight? The dilemma is that you may say you feel best at a certain weight which is above your ideal body weight. You will have to work through this and come to some conclusion. If you need to compromise with yourself, do it.

If you want to lose thirty pounds but know that you can only lose fifteen pounds effectively, do it. If you lose the entire thirty pounds and find you're not comfortable being that weight, you will start overeating again. Not only will you end up gaining all thirty pounds back, but you may find yourself gaining an additional ten pounds beyond that. Which method is more effective? Losing too much weight and then gaining it all back plus more; or losing a lesser but more reasonable amount of weight and actually keeping yourself at this reduced weight for the rest of your life?

As you get older - beyond your thirties - even if you maintain your same weight, you will lose muscle mass and actually gain fat. The weight you lose from losing muscle mass will be equal to the weight you gain from extra fat being stored on your body. To prevent this from happening, it's important to continue to work out and train your muscles to keep their bulk as you get older.

Get to a weight you feel is comfortable for you. Don't feel guilty if you don't lose all the weight you want at first. Start by losing some weight. Get exercise in addition to dieting. If you can maintain your weight loss, you'll have done yourself a great deal of good. You will find yourself feeling and looking better.

22.

Plan For Some Fun Activity In Your Day

You've been working diligently to make yourself feel and look great by utilizing all the concepts discussed so far in this book. Congratulations! Now reward yourself. Make plans for some fun activity. In fact, plan for some fun activity every day, if you can. It doesn't have to be extravagant. You don't have to travel far from your home. It can be something as simple as playing a board game, participating in a sport or allowing yourself to laugh out loud.

Even though you may enjoy working, you need to separate yourself from it. If you do nothing but work, you will ultimately burn out. You'll lose appreciation for your own talent and you'll lose site of all the other wonderful things around you as well. You will forget what makes certain things important to you. You'll lose touch with the beauty of living. All the things that you were once able to tolerate will become more irritating to you. You'll be more short-tempered and you may even stop caring about the welfare of those around you. When you end up not liking even yourself, you'll realize that you're being overwhelmed by overworking.

Although it's important to be focused on your work and career, don't let it lead you into harming yourself emotionally and physically. When you see these warning signs, you need a break. Whether it's a vacation, a good weekend of rest, a night out on the town or whatever, take it. If you need the advice of a physician, ask one. Recharge your emotional battery so you regain appreciation for, and insight into, what you do. Doing fun activities will help you gain the proper balance in your life.

When was the last time you laughed out loud? Not a polite chuckle in response to something someone said but a hearty laugh that clears out all the stress and worries in your life. This type of laughter is pure in nature and brings out a side of you that you usually repress. You must have this type of laughter in your life. There must be someone in your family, a friend, a coworker, someone on television or maybe even you yourself, who can get you laughing. Do it. When is the last time you thought of something funny and then for the rest of the day whenever you thought about it again you would laugh to yourself? This is healthy for you. Being able to laugh and thinking about the lighter side of life will benefit you greatly.

Whatever your age or your profession, you need to have fun each and every day. Having fun is a basic requirement for a complete life. Incorporating this into your life now will bring relief to your stressful and hectic day. You will feel and look great because if it.

23.

Stop Scheduling So Many Work Tasks Every Day That You Cannot Possibly Finish Them All

What's an easy way to stress yourself out? How can you make yourself feel like you're not working hard enough? How can you make yourself feel that you're falling into a bottomless pit? How can you make yourself feel that you're not doing your best at work? All of these negative things can occur if you continue to put so many work tasks on your daily schedule that you cannot possibly finish them all. This behavior leads to anxiety and a feeling of failure.

Try to organize yourself better. Be more realistic about how long tasks and projects will take. With a realistic schedule you'll still be accomplishing the same amount of work each day, but you'll appear to be more in control of the situation. Why? Because you're getting the work done you planned to do. Others around you will understand that you can accomplish what you set out to do. You'll become more of a valuable asset to others and will be thought of as a "can do" type of person. You won't have changed your work habits, you will have simply become more realistic about what you can accomplish in a single day.

In your life outside of work, you may be placing burdens on yourself that you know you can't possibly overcome. This situation leads to unnecessary stress and anxiety. There will always be matters that you cannot resolve, so accept this and know you did your best. Don't burden yourself with the emotional turmoil associated with not correcting what you set out to do. Realize that you are not superhuman.

Learn to pace yourself in your life. Don't try to accomplish so much over a weekend that when you return to work Monday morning, you feel run down and have no energy left to do the important things. It could take you the entire week to recover from overworking the previous weekend.

Stop putting so many work tasks into your plans each day when you know you can't get to all of them. If other people are depending on you to accomplish these things and they cannot be done that day, you'll only disappointment them and stress out your relationship with them. Gain control of your life. Learn to appropriate enough time to your task. If others feel you should be done sooner, tell them why you need the time and that you cannot rush. Tell them that if you're forced to rush, it may compromise your end result.

Minimize the amount of stress you place upon yourself when you schedule your day. Do everything to your best ability and don't compromise on the result. Instead of having a large daily list of things that you do poorly edit that list and do a great job on fewer things. Doing it this way will shorten the time spent correcting a bad job that may have been initially done. You will feel and look better for this.

24.

Straighten Up Your Home And Keep It That Way

If you have a neat and clean house already, congratulations! Or is your house usually cluttered, messy, unclean, even difficult to walk through because you have to navigate on small pathways through the junk you accumulate? If this sounds like your house, it's time to take action and straighten things up! If you feel your house is always messy and just isn't as nice as other people's homes, you can boost its appearance by getting rid of the mess. Throw out the junk, have a garage sale, give things away. Do whatever it takes to have your home look like a showplace again. You want to be proud of your environment.

Since you spend a lot of time in your home, you want it to have a pleasing appearance. The better the environment you can provide for yourself, the better you'll feel. Your qualities of neatness and cleanliness will not only be reflected in your home but in all aspects of your life.

Straightening up your home will immediately make it look more expensive - and the only thing you have to do is clean it up! Your house will now start to feel like the home you always wanted but felt you could never have. Remember: no matter how expensive a house is, if it's cluttered and messy, it will never look great. Maximize the appearance of your home by straightening it up and keeping it that way.

If you have created tiny pathways to walk through all the junk in your home, take inventory. You've accumulated too much and need to deal with it. Don't continue this habit. Instead, identify what you want to keep and give away the rest. Organize yourself and then take action to reclaim the space in your home. Once you clean out the junk, you'll be able to walk more freely in each room, and you'll feel like you just moved into a larger and more spacious place.

A more organized home will also appear more elegant. It will look like you redecorated. It will show that you have control over your environment. More important, you won't have to come home and see your living space looking like a battle zone. This is an easy way to regain the title "master of your domain" and it will make you feel better about yourself.

25.

Clean Out Your Car

Go out to your car and look in the window. First, is it clean enough to even see through the window? Is the interior neat or are things scattered all over so it looks like you've been driving 60 miles per hour with all the windows open? Does it look like another room in your home, so full of clutter that there's barely enough room to sit in the driver's seat? Can you identify burger wrappers and drink containers from a meal you ate weeks ago? Are there stale French fries on the car floor?

If you answer yes to these questions you can improve your car's environment. Do what's necessary to make your car look great by spending some time cleaning it up. You'll not only have more room in your car, you'll also have a greater sense of well-being because your car is clean.

Whether it's your car, your home, your office desk, your locker, all these things are important aspects of your daily life. You want to create the best environment that you can for yourself. It takes effort on your part to begin the clean up and then maintain it. But a clean and organized environment will make you feel like you're in control. Improving your surroundings will have a positive influence on you.

The environment that you live in can be made better. If it's not currently to your liking, take positive steps to change it. The best environment for you does not have to be a more expensive one. It can simply be the same one you have now, but cleaner and better organized. Make yourself feel great by cleaning up the clutter in your life!

26.

Wear Clothes That Make You Look Attractive

Go through your closet and take inventory. Reassess your clothes. Do they make you look as attractive as possibly? Do they flatter the parts of your body you know are attractive? Do they help conceal those parts of your body that are not that attractive? Do you need to place an expiration date on your clothes to let you know when it's time to make a change? If you try, you can find clothes that will make you look attractive, fit you correctly and will feel comfortable instead of feeling too tight.

When was the last time you looked in your closet to decide if your clothes are projecting the image that you want of yourself? Do you want a more professional look? A more sophisticated look? A more "with it" look? A look that makes you appear more attractive in general? Decide on the image you want and begin updating your wardrobe to represent that. Clothing is an important symbol. The clothes you wear give an immediate signal to other people about how you feel about yourself. Use this to your advantage.

Be smart about how the clothes accentuate your various body parts. Your best body attributes can be shown off with appropriately fitting clothes. If you feel your legs and arms are your best features, wear clothes which reveal them. Remember to always do this with grace and style. Show off the parts of your body you feel are positive while keeping within the accepted norms of your environment.

What about body parts that are unflattering? Use clothing to conceal them as much as possible. If you feel your hips are incredibly large compared to your upper body, wear clothing that makes you look slimmer in the hip area. For example, wear black pants instead of loud colored ones. A woman who feels her stomach is huge but her legs are thin and shapely should wear dresses that reveal her legs but minimize attention to her stomach region. If you feel your upper arms are not appealing, wear clothing to cover them. You have control over what you want to show to the rest of society.

Do you have trouble getting rid of clothes that are out of date, out of style or that simply don't make you look as attractive as you can be? Think about the concept of an expiration date for your clothes. Milk has an expiration date on the carton and everyone knows the consequences of drinking milk that has spoiled. If you cannot part with some of your old clothing, then pack it away. You may be able to use it for a Halloween costume or for a party where you dress up in clothing from a past era in your life.

Clothing that makes you look more attractive should also be comfortable to wear. In fact, the clothes that are flattering to you should be some of the most comfortable and desirable clothes you have. It will do no good to buy clothes that make you look attractive if you can't keep the pants buttoned after eating a meal. Don't get clothes that are painful to wear even if you look attractive in them. You're not helping yourself by buying inappropriate clothing. Clothing which makes you feel great to be in and makes you look your best is exactly what you want to get.

Do not settle for anything less. Do you have a pair of pants which you look great in but it is too tight in the waist? Go to the tailor and have the waist let out so you can be comfortable again. There is no reason to suffer from this. Wear clothes that make you look attractive, show off the positives, give you a sense of well being and are comfortable. You will feel and look great because of this.

27.

Get A Hairstyle That Makes You Look Attractive

Take a giant leap forward in making yourself look great by paying attention to your hairstyle. Hairstyles change over the decades, so you must be willing to reevaluate your look and change it periodically. The same hairstyle you had in high school will not look as attractive on you if you now are in your thirties. Your facial features change as you mature, so be prepared to adjust your hairstyle so you appear as attractive as possible. You don't want to look like you're lost in a hairstyle time warp. You should devote some time to your hairdo every day. Do you currently have a hairstyle that allows you to get out of the shower, let your hair dry by itself without having to work on it, and then go out in public? If this description fits, realize that your hairstyle may not be making you look as attractive as possible. People may appear unattractive simply because their hairstyles are unappealing. You want a hairstyle that is attractive and appropriate for your age and your facial features.

The proper hairstyle will make you look fabulous. Hairstyling alone can give you a great boost in your level of attractiveness. Most people need to have their hair styled professionally to accomplish this. Then you can have your hairstylist train you in how to maintain the look between your visits. If you try a new hair style and you feel it still does not make you look great, try another hairstyle or new hairstylist. It may take multiple stylings to find that look that is the most flattering to you. Once you achieve that look, go with it. You'll enjoy looking great.

Hairstyles change over the decades. If you are still wearing your hair the same you did in high school but you graduated ten or fifteen years ago, you might need to improve your look. Reevaluate your hairstyle to get the most benefit from it. If you've been out of high school for awhile, take a look through your high school year book and decide if any of those hairstyles are appropriate at this time in your life.

Be prepared to devote some time every day to maintaining an attractive hairstyle. Unless you have a styled wig that you can just pop on your head, you will have to allow yourself enough time to get your hair in shape. If you line up fifty people, half who spent time on their hair before going out and the other half who spent no time on their hair, you can usually pick out which group each person falls into. Those who spend the time to make themselves look attractive will be apparent to most observers. It's understandable if there is something happening in your life which doesn't allow you to devote time to your hair right now. But if and when you can spend the time, you'll feel better for it in the long run.

Pick a hair styling that is attractive and appropriate for your age and facial features. If a hair style looks great on someone your age but they have facial features that are different that yours, that hairstyle might not look as flattering on you. Learn to recognize this. When you look at hairstyles in magazines, try to identify people who are about your age and also have similar facial features. Look at their hairstyles more carefully because they may give you a better idea of how you will look. If you really like a hairstyling in a magazine, it may be worth trying even if you have different facial features than the model.

Remember that it may take multiple stylings to hit on a winner. Put effort into finding a hairstyle that makes you look attractive. It will also make you feel great.

28.

Switch From Glasses To Contact Lenses If You Can

Glasses can be very stylish and trendy. Some people who wear glasses don't even need their vision corrected! They wear glasses simply because they like the look the frames give them. The lenses in their glasses are clear or colored plastic and make no change to their vision. This is different than wearing glasses out of necessity. If you wear glasses to correct your vision, look at yourself in the mirror. If you have very thick glasses, the outer aspect of your face looks distorted and more narrowed when looking at your reflection through the lenses. Your eyes may look distorted and magnified and so may the wrinkles around them. The weight of the lenses may be uncomfortable. Glasses can hide your facial beauty. They can give you an aged look that is impossible to correct unless you remove your glasses or change the styling of the frames. Glasses can give you a look that you never wanted to have. They may be distorting your appearance in a way which doesn't allow you to look your best.

If you cannot switch from glasses to contact lenses, reevaluate your glasses. Can you get a frame style that allows you to look attractive? Can you get frames that make you look younger? Can you get the apparent thickness of the lens reduced? By getting smaller frames, the thicker outer part of the lens can be trimmed away in order to fit the frame without changing the way the lenses correct your vision. Get frames that complement your face and don't fight for attention when someone looks at you.

If you can switch from glasses to contact lens, do it. You can also look into the option of laser correction of your vision. After that procedure, some people no longer need glasses. If you don't want to switch from glasses completely, that's fine. You can compromise by using contacts while you are out of the house socializing or working. At home you can wear your glasses.

Glasses can hide your natural beauty. Everyone may be fixated on the glasses and not be paying attention to your facial features. No matter how much effort you put into making your face and hairstyle look as attractive as possible is may be overshadowed by your glasses.

Glasses may make you look older than you want. When people look at you, your glasses may magnify the skin around your eyes. This magnified appearance will highlight wrinkles and baggy eyelids. Many people who wear glasses don't realize that this is what others see. Switching to contacts can help reduce this effect. With contacts on or with laser eye correction, you will be able to notice the skin around your eyes more easily. Then you'll be able to do whatever is necessary to make that area look as youthful as possible.

Be careful that your glasses may give you a look that you never really wanted to create. When you look at people wearing glasses, are the glasses the first thing you notice about them? If you notice their glasses first, why is that? Are their glasses trying to create a fashion statement? Are their glasses so overpowering that you aren't able to concentrate on the conversation you're having with them? Are their glasses all you do think about? Are you noticing that they don't look their best because of their glasses? If you wear glasses, you want people to notice you first, not your glasses.

You want to look your best. If you wear glasses, are you accomplishing this? Do you need to switch your style of glasses? Can you switch to contacts or have a laser correction of your vision to reduce your need for glasses? With these things in mind, you can make yourself feel and look great.

29.

Cosmetic Makeup, If Done Properly, Can Do Wonders

Wearing cosmetic makeup can be a wonderful thing. It can boost your appearance and make your skin look better by covering up the imperfections. Makeup can give you a healthier glow so that you appear younger. It can make you feel stylish and look your best. If you have the appropriate ingredients added to your cosmetic makeup, it can also protect your skin from the sun and maximize the softness. Not only can cosmetic makeup help your skin look better at the time it's applied, it can also provide a means of caring for your skin over the long term.

You can begin by simply applying cosmetic makeup. Even if you want a natural, no-makeup look, you will need to apply the appropriate makeup to achieve that goal. You can have a natural, clean look to your skin and, at the same time, actually make it look better by using an application of light, fresh appearing cosmetics. Both men and women can benefit from using cosmetic makeup, especially to hide any skin discoloration, to conceal broken blood vessels around the nose and face and to soften the dark rings around the lower eyelids.

When you use makeup to achieve a more uniform and blended look, your appearance will improve and your skin will appear to be in better shape. Of course, makeup must be applied properly and not overdone. It should not be so intense that the only thing people notice about you is your makeup. Instead, it should complement, enhance and not distract from your appearance.

Cosmetics should give your skin a glow so that people notice your healthy coloration and assume you're taking good care of yourself. Makeup should never make you look anemic or ill. With properly applied makeup, your skin will look youthful again. You'll look like a younger version of yourself without ever having cosmetic surgery.

If you don't know how to choose the proper makeup and coloration for your skin, and aren't certain of how to best apply and blend makeup, get advice from the people at your cosmetic center. Listen to them and then pick and choose the best advice. Look at magazine photos of people about your age whose facial features and coloration are similar to yours. Look carefully and identify which makeup makes them look better and which distracts from their looks. Use those products and techniques that will make you look your best.

The wonderful thing about cosmetic makeup is that other ingredients are added to the product that can do wonders for your skin. These things can provide you with proper skin care, which is necessary for the rest of your life. For example, always get a makeup that contains a sunblock, designated by a SPF (Sun Protection Factor) number. The higher the SPF number, the better the protection. If you can find an SPF of 45 or higher, that's great! Just be aware that the sunblock available in cover makeup is not always as high as what you can get in a regular bottle of suntan lotion. Sunblock is especially important during the sunny months of the year and if you go on a warm sun vacation. It's also good to use sunblock when you go snow skiing because snow reflects a lot of sunlight. The sunblock in your makeup will protect you from getting a sunburn. It'll help reduce premature aging, wrinkling of the skin, the incidence of precancerous skin changes and skin cancers, all of which can be caused by sunburns.

Cosmetic makeup should also have an alpha hydroxy acid (AHA) in it. The alpha hydroxy acid acts as a skin exfoliant which helps soften the skin. The alpha hydroxy acid will not eliminate wrinkles but it will give your skin a better overall texture. The alpha hydroxy acids are naturally occurring acids found in many things including sugar cane, milk and apples. Glycolic acid is a common type of alpha hydroxy acid derived from sugar cane. The concentration of the alpha hydroxy acid in makeup is low enough, 2% to 8%, that you can apply it daily. If you notice too much skin irritation from the alpha hydroxy acid you may need to reduce the concentration you apply. The alpha hydroxy acid also acts as a sunblock but it has an SPF value of only 2.5.

If the concentration of the alpha hydroxy acid were a lot higher, 25% to 50% concentration, you would not be able to tolerate daily applications for the rest of your life. It would be too irritating to your skin. Only a doctor can apply high concentrations of an alpha hydroxy acid to your skin, usually once a week for up to six to eight weeks. The doctor will leave the alpha hydroxy acid on the skin for only several minutes each time but will increase the concentration weekly. The skin is allowed to recover between treatments.

If you use a moisturizer before you apply your makeup, you will condition your skin to allow the alpha hydroxy acid to penetrate even deeper and further maximize its result. The manufacturer may add other ingredients to the makeup to improve skin.

Cosmetic makeup, if applied properly, can make you look great. It's a wonderful addition to your daily life, so use it every day and not just on special occasions. Your skin will look much better the moment you apply the makeup. With the addition of special ingredients, cosmetic makeup will protect your skin and add to its youthful appearance for years to come.

30.

Carry Yourself With Pride

Hold your head up high and your back straight. Be proud of yourself and carry yourself in a way that's classy and stylish. Understand that you should be proud of who and what you are. You don't need to be anyone else; you can be yourself. Feel on the inside that you are proud of yourself and it will reflect on your outward appearance. Don't let yourself be influenced by any put-downs others may have given you. You'll be able to put up a mental force field to block unkind remarks and not let it affect you. In fact, doing so will make you stronger. You must remember to be true to yourself.

By holding your head high and back straight, you are doing the outward things which in turn give you more inner strength and pride. This positive body language sets you apart from all the others around you. When you see other people carrying themselves with pride, you will immediately recognize it. Without even speaking to those people you already have visual clues as to what type of individuals they are. Their inner selves are projected onto their outer selves like a motion picture on a giant movie screen theater.

Understand the basic good within you. You will win out over all the evil that may be surrounding you. Be yourself. Don't spend all your time worrying about trying to be someone else. If you find a trait you like in another person, take action so you can emulate this trait yourself. Keep working at it. You have the skill and ability to be the very person you want to be.

Make the effort to continue to grow and develop. Be true to yourself; no one else can do it for you. Feel the pride. You will look better when others see you. Appreciate all the good you can do in this world - it makes you who you are. Carry yourself with pride because it will help you feel and look great.

31.

Walk With Confidence

Walk with confidence in your life. Even if you don't feel you should walk with confidence, do it anyway. Regardless of your level of confidence, start now and project that feeling. If you have a disability that prevents you from walking as you desire, you can still express yourself with confidence. Build up your confidence as you would build up your muscle strength through exercising. Take your confidence with you in your stride and apply it to all the other aspects of your life.

Have confidence in yourself. Start with simple things, gain confidence and build from there. Begin by learning to make a simple yes or no decision. Become more confident in your decisions and you'll see that you will trust yourself even more. Your decisions will become more beneficial to you and will lead you in the right direction. If you know that you cannot, at the present time, make a decision on a particular matter because of its complexity, have the confidence to acknowledge this very fact. You also need to be able to say you're not ready to make your decision. Your confidence will aid you in the entire process of decision-making.

Building up your level of confidence is an ongoing process. Events continually happen that threaten to shatter your confidence. Your belief in yourself is always being tested. Have the strength, courage and endurance to continue being confident. Stand up to the challenge. It's a lifelong process that will help you grow and develop.

Begin with simple tasks you can manage. Each time you accomplish these tasks, you gain confidence in yourself. Any complex task or challenge you will face is only a group of simple tasks strung together. Never imagine resolving a complex task in one motion. It makes it seem too difficult. Break down the challenge in front of you into a string of more simple tasks. Do them one at a time and you'll ultimately complete what seemed impossible.

Your confidence should extend to all aspects of your life. If you find yourself with the confidence at work to get the job done, take that feeling and apply it to the other areas of your life that you'd like to strengthen. It will assist you in accomplishing things you want to do. Walk with confidence. You will feel better and look better because of it.

32.

Treat Others As You Would Want To Be Treated Yourself

How do you want to be treated? Do you want to be treated with respect? Do you want others to listen to you when you speak? Do you want people to be polite to you when you interact with them? Do you want others to be respectful of your personal belongings? Do you want others to call you back on the phone when you leave them a message to do so? Do you want others to have a kind word to say to you? Would you like to be greeted by other people with smiles on their faces? Would you like to have a door held open for you when you are walking in with your hands full? You obviously have answered yes to these questions. You want to be treated well by others in all aspects of your life.

The best way to ensure that others treat you well is to make certain you're treating other people well. Treat others as you would want to be treated yourself. Your demeanor and character will show through and people will be more willing to take the step to treat you better. If you learn to make eye contact with them and smile, you're much more likely to interact with others in a positive way.

If you want someone to be polite to you, the best way to accomplish this is to be polite to them when you're talking. If one person starts off a conversation by not being polite, then the other person falls into the trap of thinking they must also be impolite in the same conversation. This is a bad habit to form.

Do not allow others to change your personality into something you don't want it to be. There are always situations where, no matter how well mannered you are, you will encounter extremely rude people.

The best practice is to always show respect for everyone. You will not have to try to remember if you treated others well or badly when you make their re-acquaintance. Treat everyone with respect and you won't have to act differently around different individuals.

To make yourself feel great treat others as you would want to be treated. You'll be more pleasant and it will be easier for you to interact with others. You'll be less stressed because every encounter you have with someone will not have to be a battle. Your facial expressions will be more relaxed and you will find yourself frowning less.

33.

Volunteer Your Time To Something That Makes You Feel Good About Yourself

Giving of yourself is an uplifting feeling - whether it's for an established organization or on your own. By volunteering your time, you can lend your talents and abilities to others for a good cause. You can volunteer once a week, once a month, once a year, whatever you can fit into your schedule. It should be a win-win situation for both yourself and the people you are helping. If you do not feel good about volunteering for a particular cause, you'll find yourself dropping the project before very long. In order to honor your commitment as a volunteer, choose causes and activities that are personally fulfilling.

You'll feel good because you've volunteered. Those feelings of joy, importance and self worth are good things to experience. They'll help you grow and develop in your personal life. Volunteering is the right thing to do. Even though you don't get paid for your services, you'll receive personal rewards that are more valuable than money.

Established organizations such as hospitals, churches and schools are always in need of volunteers. They already have specific ongoing activities already established that you can help with. You can also create your own volunteer activity. If there is some area you feel is deficient in volunteerism, you can correct this situation. You may feel that your community doesn't know enough about something that should be important to everyone. If you're extremely knowledgeable about that subject, you could help educate people by giving free lectures in your community center or in the public library meeting room.

If you have unique talents and abilities, volunteering them may be an even more valuable gift to give others. If you're a master at the computer, it may be more valuable to teach others how to improve their computer skills for an hour instead of spending that time simply stuffing envelopes. Although stuffing envelopes may be a critical activity to keep the volunteer organization running smoothly, you should still try to provide your best talents when you volunteer.

How often you volunteer is based on how often the organization needs your help and how often you are available to provide your services. Some great causes may only need help once a year. Other causes may need help on a weekly basis. Work out a schedule you can manage. Pace yourself and do not initially overcommit. If you overburden yourself at the start, you may burn out quickly. You don't want to make yourself quit volunteering.

A win-win situation is what you desire related to you volunteering. If it's not good for both yourself and the people you're helping, there's something wrong with the situation. In a win-win situation you are more likely to want to continue to provide help. The people you help will be thankful and you'll understand why you're volunteering in the first place. It will keep you invigorated. Volunteering should fill you with a positive emotion that will help keep you coming back to help.

Doing something that's personally fulfilling and helps others is a wonderful thing to do. To volunteer yourself to a cause is a great thing. Everyone should benefit from it. You'll make yourself feel great because you are a volunteer.

34.

Look In The Mirror To See If You Are Going In The Right Direction

Take inventory of yourself by looking in the mirror. Do you see yourself going in the right direction? Turn this into a positive, and not a negative, situation. You can control the direction your life is heading. You have the ability and talent to carry this out. It's important to reevaluate where you're at in your life. You have to decide if you're doing things that are helpful or hurtful. Eliminate the hurtful things and get yourself back on the right course. It does help to look in the mirror and see yourself in this way.

When you look in the mirror, think about your outward appearance and your inner self. They are dependent on each other and it's equally important for you to take care of both. It will be to your benefit to do so.

Make this self-evaluation a positive, and not a negative, experience. Having the ability to identify and then work through a problem should be viewed as a positive skill. Use this skill to make yourself a better and stronger person. You'll soon realize that fixing and correcting things are more easily accomplished. Once you think of yourself as a problem solver, you'll have less anxiety about it.

You should now understand that you have the ability and talent to accomplish change. You are the one who is most responsible for yourself. Be proud of this fact. It's you, not someone else, who can take the first step in the right direction. You don't have to wait to see if someone else will or will not allow you to do it. You don't have to wait to see if someone else needs to finish their agenda first. You can do the positive things without being delayed by other people.

To make yourself feel and look great you have to steer yourself in the right direction in life. It doesn't happen by chance or luck or from neglect on your part. It requires your active participation. The more you take the lead, the better off you'll be.

35.

Having A Pet At Home Can Lift Your Mood

Why do we often see television clips of dogs being brought into nursing homes and pediatric wards at hospitals? It's done because it's felt that dogs will lift the spirits of those who hold and play with them. It's hoped the patients will forget about their problems or how bad they might be feeling. It's understood that pets have a wonderful power over us – a power to brighten our lives and make us feel better about ourselves.

If you're able to get a pet, if you have the room for it and if you can care for it, a pet would be a great addition to your family. Don't fool yourself though, there's always work to be done because of a pet. You must be willing to understand this and not get frustrated at your pet because of it. A new pet is a lot like a new baby in the family. A pet requires attention, caring for and grooming. It must be taken to the veterinarian to maintain its health. A pet also must be housebroken.

Though new pets are work, they also are cuddly, cute, and fun to be with. Pets provide hours of pure laughter and are a blessing. As your new pet improves on his or her manners and is more house-friendly, it will be even easier living with your pet. What a pet will add to your family's well-being cannot be measured. A pet makes you realize the simpler joys in life. Throwing a rubber toy and watching your dog run after it, pick it up, come back to you and then try to prevent you from taking the toy out of its mouth is a simple and fun game. It doesn't require a lot of thought. It's enjoyable interaction at its most basic level.

Lift your spirits over the long term and get a pet. Gain all the benefits that others have gained from having a pet at home. It may remind you of all those pleasant memories you had of your childhood pet. You'll remember how important your pet was to you and the rest of your family. You'll remember how you would take your pet for a walk. And you'll recall how your pet never seemed to get tired even though you would spend hours playing together.

Having a pet will brighten your life and make you feel better about yourself. The burdens you bring home from work will be left at the door step as soon as your pet comes running up to you. You won't have time to sulk over events of the day because your mind and efforts will be occupied playing with your pet. A pet will never complain, tell you if it thinks you're mean or tell you anything negative. Your pet is always happy to see you and be with you.

Feel great by getting yourself a pet. Your pet will help you be more calm. You are likely to be at ease more often. Troubling things may start to bother you less. You'll appreciate the simple joys in life as you enjoy your pet.

36.

Stay Away From People Who Make You Feel Bad

It's not always clear why other people want to make you feel bad about yourself. Is it family members, co-workers, bosses, customers or other people you run into who do this to you? They may be acting out of envy or jealousy. They may be trying to make themselves feel superior and you, inferior. They may know perfectly well that they are trying to make you feel bad about yourself or they're so clueless that they do not realize what's happening. It's not hard to tell the difference between this behavior and constructive criticism. Negative people create situations where the only purpose of their conversation with you or their actions toward you is to make you feel bad about yourself. It's important to learn to avoid these sorts of people and situations.

It's not necessary for you to get into the minds of those who make you feel bad. You just need to identify who these people are and do your best to minimize your exposure to them. In this way you can reduce the unnecessary attacks on you. Remember: they are the ones who have a problem, not you. You should not allow them to destroy your perfectly good day. These people represent only a minority of all the people you come in contact with each day and you must learn not to allow them to monopolize your thoughts. Don't dwell on the bad things they say to you or how much they hurt your feelings. Realize what they do to you and work on getting negative thought out of your head immediately. Each time their negativity drifts back into your thoughts, think about something else.

What if you're in a situation where you can't minimize your exposure to these people? It may be a family member whom you can't avoid or a customer or boss with whom you are in daily contact. You may have to be honest with these people. You may have to tell them that you welcome constructive criticism but they must stop saying negative things that are only hurtful to you.

Others may try to make themselves feel superior to you. They want you to feel bad, but don't fall into their trap. They are playing a game in which they should be the only player. Leave yourself out of their game.

Again, these are not the majority of people you encounter. They are few in number but they have the most negative impact on you. It may take you days to recover from their verbal bashings. You, in turn, may feel so hurt that you treat others around you badly. Unfortunately, you then perpetuated those feelings of negativity too long and to other people. Learn how to stop this from happening.

You can make yourself feel and look great. If you can't avoid these negative people, learn how to deal with them quickly. The fact that you can identify them is a plus. Realize what they are trying to do to you and take action against their negativity.

Previously in this book you learned how to rid yourself of a negative thought and go on with your day. Your own mood with be lightened and you won't have a strained look on your face. You'll look better in the mirror. Your smile will make other people happy and you'll be much better off too.

37.

Relearn The Art Of Conversation By Allowing Only One Person To Speak At A Time

Our society is leading us away from effective communication. On television and radio we are unfortunately learning that it is acceptable not to allow others to speak out in a full sentence. You see time and again how someone is interrupted in mid-sentence by another person trying to voice his or her own opinion. People are not being allowed to complete a thought. One annoying strategy involves shouting and trying to drown out the initial speaker's voice in order to grab attention. You probably have encountered situations where everyone starts speaking at the same time. There may be four people together, each speaking out with no one listening. The one who finally gets attention and the speaking floor is the one who simply keeps talking while everyone else finally stops due to exhaustion. It's like an endurance race - if you can't keep up the pace of constantly talking you never get a chance to speak.

Establish the ground rules when you're with others. Let them know you want to listen to what they're saying but they must also be willing to listen to you. Relearn the lost art of conversation. Allowing one person to speak at a time is a good way to start this process. You learn much more from listening to others than you ever learn from listening to yourself speak.

The next time you turn on the television or the radio or are out in public, listen carefully when two people begin discussing an issue. Are you having trouble understanding what they are saying because they keep interrupting each other? If they interrupt each other constantly, each person probably feels he or she can only win the conversation by not allowing the other to speak. It is important for you to identify this behavior and not make the same mistake. When you're with others, listen to what they have to say. Listening is a skill that requires effort on your part. Allow people to finish their train of thought before you speak. Others will view you as being intelligent because you have the ability to listen. In order to become intelligent one must be willing to listen and learn.

Take charge the next time your conversation is being lost by interruptions. Let everyone know what's happening. Lead by your example and teach others how to have a productive conversation with you. You'll feel better when you have your next talk with someone. It will feel more effortless. You'll have a whole new outlook because you no longer have to concern yourself with how to interrupt the other person. You have relearned the art of conversation.

38.

Get Started Now On These Suggestions, Don't Wait Until A Year From Now

Don't wait for one year to go by before you get started making yourself feel and look great. Get started now! Don't allow any more time to pass without doing anything. You know what you have to do and there's no excuse for putting it off any longer. Think of all that you can gain personally from this book over a one-year period. At the end of one year you'll look back and be grateful that you started. If you do absolutely nothing from this book and reassess yourself in one year, you'll realize you could have bettered yourself but did not. Challenge yourself to make a go of it this time!

These suggestions are not meant to be utilized for a brief period of time and then forgotten. To have the maximum benefit they must become part of your way of life. It makes the most sense to be consistent because the more consistent you are, the more likely it is that you'll see the benefits you've gained. You'll be able to look back to where you started and see what a true accomplishment you've made.

By following this book's suggestions, you'll turn yourself into a "can-do" person. The totality of life is broken down into its more recognizable components so each suggestion is manageable because it involves only a small part of your life. The areas you want to improve are begging for you to get started. Some of these suggestions don't entail any hard work; they only involve the way you look at yourself or at other people or things. For the ones that do involve working up a sweat, have fun with them!

Don't take one giant leap forward in one single moment. You may not reach what you seek. Instead, take small steps, consistent steps, safe steps, reproducible steps, steps in the correct direction to get to your next level. You want to grow more confident and be able to reproduce your success again and again. To improve your tennis game, you wouldn't take one lesson and then go out to play your next game expecting to be vastly improved. You have to keep working on what you learned and improving your skills. As the weeks, months and years go by, you can look back at where you started and understand how better you're playing over the long run. You didn't achieve maximum benefit from your lesson at the very beginning. You had to incorporate it into your play and use it again and again. Take this attitude and approach life in this way.

Many professions require years of training for a person to achieve the skill and understanding that is required to practice that profession. Think of making yourself feeling and looking great as a profession. You have to spend the time and energy to reach a professional level. It also requires ongoing reassessment and reeducation to maintain the level you will achieve.

How can you make yourself feel and look great? Get started with the suggestions that have been laid out here. There may be things not mentioned in this book that you feel can help you improve yourself. Identify these things and what you need to accomplish them. Go forward with them. Feeling and looking great is but a small step away!

39.

Smile And Laugh

Express joy in your life. A smile and laughter bring you closer to this. A smile is also is a polite way to acknowledge the presence of another person. You always look better with a smile than with a frown. You look more youthful and your appearance is brighter when you smile. Laughter, when appropriate, has a calming effect. It helps you forget about the daily stresses in your life and puts you in a better mood. Smiling and laughing help you feel and look better.

A smile can immediately establish a positive interaction with someone. It is a nonverbal form of communication that can be as important as what you actually say. A healthy relationship can result from a smile. It can be your ally. If you aren't smiling, are you frowning? A frown sends a nonverbal signal to others that you're unhappy to be around them, that you're not feeling well or that you're personally unhappy. The wrong facial expression can wipe out anything you verbally say to people. They may not believe what you're saying because of your facial signals.

Laughter always will be what it is - a simple way to express yourself when something is funny or amusing. It is easily contagious. If others are laughing, you may start laughing too even though you don't know why. A difficult day may seem less overwhelming when you add laughter to it. Looking at the lighter side of an issue that is concerning you can bring out laughter. This ability to laugh in the face of high stress is a necessary release. You can't continue with a glum look on your face for the rest of your life. Laughter can put you back on track with reality. Don't let the issues you face in life overtake your thoughts and emotions and prevent you from laughing. Don't lose sight of the importance of laughter and its ability to cleanse away the worries that have been clinging to you.

You must even add laughter to some of your most stressful life experiences. It will help you understand that life can and does goes on and that tomorrow can be a better day for you. Laughter gives you a ray of hope to go forward. It is extremely therapeutic and may have as much effect on you as the medicine you take. The end result of laughing may be that you forget why you were so concerned in the first place. Laughter is important in our life. *Reader's Digest* magazine has a section called "Laughter is the Best Medicine." When you talk out your troubles with others, you'll also find that you're not alone in your worries. Everyone else around you may be experiencing similar difficulties. You can find laughter in this common bond.

A comedian said when he was in China, which has a population of over one billion people, someone told him he was "one in a million." To that he said, "You mean I'm just like a thousand other guys?"

Smiling and laughing are important and powerful. Incorporate them into your life. They can get you through a difficult day or make a good day even better. They can help you to interact more easily with others. A smile will make you look your best. And laughter makes you feel your finest.

40.

Read Other Books On Self Help

The more information you're exposed to the more knowledge you'll gain. Other books, CD's and videos are available to improve yourself. Look these over and decide if you can gain anything from them. You may disagree with them on some points and agree on other points. Extract whatever useful information they have to offer you.

Expanding your knowledge base leads to personal growth which leads to self-improving. With more knowledge you may reach a point where things start to look less black-and-white and fall more into zones of gray. Conflicting information may start to overwhelm you. Don't be fearful of this, just realize that you've reached a high level of understanding. Don't fall into the trap of not doing anything that can help you because you've been confused and neutralized by conflicting information.

Other sources of information are also useful to examine. You may have a certain perspective on yourself and the way to live your life. It should be interesting to see from your readings if others share your perspective or not. It's also interesting to see how other people propose a solution to a problem you may already be working on.

There's always something to be gained by continuing to read about personal improvement. You may read something that you never considered in the past that further enlightens you. Small bits of information or better ways to look at something may come your way.

You are on the proper path so continue your education into feeling and looking great. It's a terrific, fun road to travel! It is for your benefit. New insight is there for the taking around each bend in the road. Keep it up!

41.

Surround Yourself With Beautiful And Elegant Things

Feel fortunate if you are able to have beautiful and elegant things surround you. It's an uplifting experience, so take advantage of it. Your environment can provide you with inspiration, feelings of well-being and a true appreciation of your surroundings. If you don't have these kinds of things in your own home, you can go to an art store, visit a museum or walk through a beautiful park or neighborhood. Study the local architecture in your community. Visit an area that makes you feel good about yourself.

Walking through an area with fascinating architecture is a delight. Notice how a building's form and landscaping can affect your mood. If you're in a down mood, stroll through a beautiful area and see how much better you feel at the end of the walk. You can appreciate the fact that others have dedicated their lives to creating things of beauty for everyone to enjoy.

Walk though a garden and really look at the flowers. Their shapes and colors will reawaken your understanding of what exquisite things can be found on this earth. Don't shut beautiful and elegant things out of your life. They are meant to be cherished and embraced for your benefit.

During my college years at Brown University, an Ivy League institution in Providence, Rhode Island; I would take walks through the campus and the surrounding neighborhoods. These walks weren't intended to get me from one place to another. They simply allowed me to look at and feel the beauty of the architecture around me. The memorable inscriptions I read on the cornerstones of building erected centuries ago were delightful. From the inscriptions I realized people throughout history have a passion for who they were, what they did and what they believed in.

Studying such inscriptions makes the lives of these people and their accomplishments even more meaningful. One inscription cited the virtues of strength, courage and endurance in order to make yourself invincible. The strength referred to is mental as well as physical strength. Courage involves continuing on your path no matter what the obstacles confront or discourage you. The virtue of endurance underscores the fact that you do not and cannot become who you are in a split second. This is a process which requires time. To be able to grow and mature takes endurance.

Walking along a river, a pond, a lake or ocean front can be a breathtaking event. The sound of the water running past you can be hypnotic. The gentleness of the waves and the shapes they assume as they fall onto the shore is inviting. Immeasurable beauty surrounds you on this earth.

Make yourself feel great by taking the time to look at and appreciate all the beautiful and elegant things around you. If you have to explore your own house or neighborhood to find these things, do so. You may be surprised to discover them directly outside your window and to learn that you were just too preoccupied before to have seen them for what they really are.

42.

Reach For The Heavens

Set your goals high. Don't think you are incapable of doing wonderful things. Do your best and even if you fall short you have still gained much. There is no reason to put a mental restriction on what you may attain in your future. You are the one who can reach for the heavens. You are the one to make the decision to proceed with achieving your goals. You will feel great knowing you have this type of power within you.

If you set your goals too low, once you've achieved them you'll start to feel bored and unchallenged. You'll then need to reestablish your goals and make them higher, more challenging and more interesting. Even great explorers find other challenges to conquer once they've reached their original goal. Getting through college can be a great challenge. Once you graduate you go out to utilize your education to do even greater things. You may take on a job or pursue graduate or professional education. Many of the goals you've achieved can be considered steps up to even higher levels of self-accomplishment. Each small step is important and lays the foundation for who you are.

Don't think that you're unable to do great things. The only thing that may separate you from someone who's achieved something wonderful is that they took the action to achieve it and you have not yet taken that step. So set your goal and take the necessary action. Once you've achieved your goal, you'll look back and tell yourself you were always capable of it.

You won't be able to reach every goal you set. But if you don't take action, you'll never know how close you would have come. By falling short you've still won because you've allowed yourself to grow and develop. You must be proud of yourself and not consider yourself a failure. Others will look at what you've done and won't be able to understand why you're down on yourself. Learn to accept the fact that you can succeed just by trying.

Don't erect mental barriers as to what you can achieve in your life. In the free society in which we exist, we don't have to accept these barriers. Don't place restrictions on yourself. Free your mind. Don't clutter your thoughts with things that you tell yourself you cannot do. Put those things that you want to do into your head and take action.

Don't measure yourself based only on how much money you have. You can always find someone who has more money than you do. Instead, measure yourself on the basis of the type of person you are, what you mean to others and what you have to offer society.

You are the one with the power to reach for the heavens. Do it! Don't put yourself down or restrict yourself. Don't feel that it's always the other person and not you who can succeed. It's your time to shine. You must take action to reach for the heavens. You'll be proud of yourself and feel great.

43.

Get Into A Groove

Become productive at both work and play. You can call this "getting into a groove." Everything will feel like it is moving forward and going right. Professional athletes call this "being in a zone." You'll find that you're accomplishing a lot in your professional career and having a lot of fun with your leisure time. Some of your best work may be ahead of you if you can get yourself into a groove or zone and go with it. Athletes will have some of their highest scoring games at these times. A basketball player may feel the basketball hoop looks ten times bigger than it usually does so that it's suddenly easier to shoot the basketball and score.

To baseball batters who are in a groove, a pitched ball appears as a giant beach ball slowly floating directly over home plate toward them. They may hit the ball for a home run or simply make great contact with the ball and get on base.

Tennis players who are at this heightened level will feel like they're ballet dancers moving gracefully from one side of the court to the other with seemingly no effort at all. They hit the ball easily because it appears to them much bigger than it really is. It seems to be moving in slow motion and is easier to see. They sense the racket has a will of its own to make solid contact with the ball every time.

A business person who's in a zone may find it much easier than expected to write a manual on office procedures. The ability to generate the ideas for the necessary chapters may seem effortless. The words may flow out of their head as fast as water over a waterfall.

On the job you may take only two hours to complete the same amount of work that took you four hours on another day. The time difference won't be caused by interruptions that delayed your progress, but by the fact you were in a groove or zone. This enabled you to work more effectively and quickly. The exact same tasks were simply easier to do.

The common denominator in each of these experiences is a heightened state of mind. Everything appears much clearer and more obvious than usual, as though you've put on corrective glasses and sharpened your focus on the tasks at hand. At these times you'll appear to do everything with very little effort even though you're actually working very hard. You'll be extremely focused on the matter at hand and won't be bothered by any distractions around you.

Get into a groove or zone in your life. If you don't know how, then learn to identify when you have spontaneously gotten into a groove. This is when you should do some of your greatest work because it will seem easy to you. You'll feel great knowing the level of focus you can achieve and how it can benefit you.

44.

Never Stop The Learning Process

Never stop the learning process. It's more than just listening to someone telling you something. You may have completed your formal education many years ago and thought that you had learned everything there was to know. Several years later you probably realized that learning doesn't just stop. No matter where you are currently in life, always view education as an ongoing phenomenon. Do this and you'll be forever grateful. You'll feel great knowing that you will continue to educate yourself. You may want to pursue knowledge at your local library, at home, or on the Internet. Go wherever you want to find the appropriate resources to study and learn from.

During my medical school education we had full days of lectures. The lectures were meant to familiarize everyone with the information which needed to be learned. So why did all the medical students still spent hours at the library after class studying and memorizing? Simply because no one could retain all that new information just by listening to it one time in the classroom. In order to absorb the new information, students had to study and review it.

Accept the fact that you can't always learn and understand something based on hearing it only once. Realize that no one is able to retain the information in his or her head after listened to it a single time. True learning and understanding occurs during the hours of studying in the library or at home. You not only learn facts, you also come to appreciate the concepts involved. This makes the facts easier to understand.

You'll be happy that you've continued the learning process. Think about the changes you've made in your own work. The way you did things in the past may have become outdated and less efficient. You changed with the times because you knew it would benefit you and your work. You allowed yourself to learn and understand new and better ways of doing things. In a decade you may be doing your work in a way you wouldn't think was possible now. Technology will exist that you can't even imagine at this time. You'll want to be involved with these ongoing innovations. Develop the habit of continuing your education. Learning and incorporating new things into your life should become part of your daily routine.

If you need the formal setting of a library to continue to educate yourself, go there. If you can do this from your home or at work, that's fine too. You may have multiple locations you enjoy to go to and feel comfortable in when you study. You want to be in a mood that allows you to concentrate on the subject matter. The resources you choose to learn from are also important. Seek out sources that make it easy and fun for you to learn. Make sure they allow you to see the overall picture of what you're learning. Allow yourself to learn for the rest of your life. You'll enjoy the personal growth and development that results from expanding your mind.

45.

Take A Relaxing Shower

There are many benefits to taking a relaxing shower. Water has such a therapeutic effect that you'll feel good just knowing you're headed to the shower. Once the water hits, you will benefit from both its soothing effect and its invigorating force. You'll be reawakened and your entire body will feel like it's had a massage. You'll be ready to face the rest of the day. Spending time in the shower will get you in a good mood because it's time you truly spend on yourself.

People have known about the therapeutic effect of running water for thousands of years. They've sought out and gone into streams to nurse their sore or ailing body back to health. Animals instinctively seek out and wade in running water to make themselves feel better. Athletes who injure their legs sit in a tank of rapidly circulating water for up to half an hour each day until they recover from their injuries. Running water on your body can be very beneficial but you don't need to seek out a river or go to a college athletic facility. You can use a home whirlpool if you have one, use the whirlpool at your health club or simply take a shower.

Heading to the shower can be a fun ritual. You'll feel good just anticipating what the shower will do for you. It's similar to the joy you experience before you go on vacation. Even though you have not left for the trip yet, you feel wonderful knowing that you're going away soon. Taking a shower is like a vacation from the distractions in your life.

Water soothes your mind. A shower can wash away your troubles and concerns and help refocus your thoughts on more pleasurable things. You may not even be aware this is happening, but it does occur. A shower also invigorates you in a positive way. It helps you feel better about yourself and what you're capable of doing. If you've had a bad day at work, jump into the shower as soon as you get home. When you walk out of the shower, you'll find you've forgotten why it was such a bad day in the first place.

A shower can feel like an entire body massage because in the process of washing your body, you've also massaged your skin and muscles. It's as if a professional masseuse made a personal visit to your house. You're in touch with your physical self and your body is reawaked. If you get out of bed early in the morning and don't know how you're going to make it through the rest of the day, try taking a shower. After your shower you may decide that the day is there just for your personal benefit.

Taking a relaxing shower is a great mood-altering device. It's a simple, natural way to change how you feel. So make yourself feel and look great by taking a relaxing shower.

46.

Enjoy The Moment At Hand

Don't wait until some time in the future to enjoy life, do it now! Don't allow worry to prevent you from enjoying the present. Enjoy the fact that you're reading this book and helping yourself because of it. Enjoy the free time you're giving yourself to further expand your mental boundaries. Enjoy your ability to see, feel and hear the world in which you live. Enjoy the fact that you have the capability to be the person you want to be. Enjoy those who are close to you. Realize that there are many wonderful things you can enjoy in your life right now.

There is no time like the present time to enjoy yourself. If you can't start to enjoy life now, how do you think that you'll be able to at some future time? What will be so different about your life that you can finally take joy in it? Learn to enjoy the present. If you do, you can predict that in the future you'll also be enjoying your life because each future day quickly becomes the present.

You can always find something to worry about in your life. You may be able to resolve those things that are currently an issue but there will always be some other issue to worry about. You can't let these worries prevent you from enjoying your life. Current and future problems will always confront you. Maybe you're telling yourself that you can't enjoy life right now because of certain family matters that are bothering you. You promise that as soon as these troubling family matters go away, you can get back on track with enjoying yourself. But as soon as you free yourself from these worries, you'll be surprised to find that another crisis has developed. Then you're telling yourself that you can't enjoy life until the new crisis is resolved.

Life is a series of ongoing crises. You must learn to enjoy life now though you may be surrounded by unfortunate events. Learn this and you'll appreciate the present and enjoy life for what it is. Life is also a series of both predictable and unpredictable events. How you conduct yourself in the present will influence how positively or negatively those events affect you. Be strong so the events in your life will shape your personality in a positive way.

Take simple pleasure in being able to appreciate the words in this book. Your ability to read and understand is a wonderful thing. Sitting down and concentrating only on what you're reading can bring great joy. You can be totally immersed in a book but still come up safely for air. When you read, you expand the limits of your comprehension and catapult yourself into previously unrealized territories. You'll land unharmed and be all the better for it.

Enjoy the moment at hand. There are people and things in your life at the present time that you will remember forever. Appreciate the fact that they are in your life now. Enjoy your time spent with them. Enjoy what life has to offer you and you will feel and look better.

47.

Learn To Get Yourself Motivated

Being motivated about something is an emotional high that allows you to focus your energy on achieving something and being productive. You need to understand what motivates you so that you can learn to motivate yourself now and in the future. Words spoken by another person can energize you. You may find motivation in a specific paragraph in a specific book you have read. Being around other people may motivate you. Or you may motivate yourself by remembering something outstanding that you did in the past.

Becoming energized is very emotional. You have to get yourself psyched up about what you want to do. Once you're psyched up, you'll find you have the inspiration to carry yourself forward with the work or project at hand. Having inspiration is like having a giant locomotive train pushing 100 box cars that are at rest. The locomotive will push and get the boxcars going at full speed in no time. Without the help of the locomotive, the boxcars would not have gotten anywhere. It's important to have passion about what you are doing. Don't just walk into a situation without emotion. Take your feelings and incorporate them into your tasks in a positive way.

With the momentum of a mental push, you'll discover that you are able to be highly productive. That push or shove is meant to get you started but the energy you need is already there. A project you've put off for a long time can now be approached. Think of your mind as a pilot light on a stove. To get all the energy and effort you need, you simply turn the dial up and get a full flame to appear.

Understanding what motivates you can be used to your advantage. You can generate the spark you need to accomplishment something. You have the control to initiate what others may find difficult to do. Tasks may appear easier to you even though they may be challenging. You can discard your mental barriers against what you used to be afraid of trying.

Do the spoken words of others motivate you? Can you recall what those words are? Do you repeat those words in your head again and again to do the trick of motivating yourself? Has someone paid you such a great complement that every time you think about what they said, you get so energized that you want to stand up on your feet and get started on any job in front of your?

Have you read something in the past which you feel is truly inspiring? Every time you recall the story, do your emotional juices start to flow? Does it cause you to want to take action? Do you feel like you've tapped into an exhilarating source of energy?

Are there people you've personally met or seen in the media whom, by their actions or their accomplishments, you find exceptionally inspiring? Understand that it's good to have heroes in your life. Such people and what they can do or have done should be emulated. The positive influence they can have on you is tremendous. Think about them to help get yourself motivated.

A negative event from the past may inspire you now. If something occurred and ever since then you've told yourself, "I'm never going to let that happen again", you're energizing yourself with that thought. Your own outstanding past actions can also be a great catalyst. You can recall a wonderful thing you did and the effort it took to accomplish it. You'll find inspiration in this past action that will allow you to take action again. You will feel great knowing you have the ability to motivate yourself.

48.

Learn To Be Patient

Everything you want may not come to you instantly. Certain things have to be earned through persistent effort. You must be able to recognize what these things are and be patient about receiving them. Learning to be patient will give you a great perspective on self-gratification. You'll understand that there is a time and place for everything and that you may not be rewarded for your labor at this exact moment in time. It may occur well after you thought it would happen. That is the difference between instant and delayed gratification.

What sorts of things can't come to you instantly? If you're pursuing a higher level of education like college or professional schooling, you know that all the learning and experience you'll need can't be attained in a week. It will take years for you to learn before you graduate. If you're taking a three-month course at your community college on how to improve your skills on the computer, don't expect to understand everything after a few classes. You must give yourself the full allotted time in order to learn and understand the material.

If you're exercising to get in shape, you know that a single day of working out won't get you to your desired level of fitness. It may take weeks, months or longer to reach your goal. You still, however, receive immediate satisfaction and feel great for having started your workout program.

You may have altered your diet today so you would eat the proper food to lose weight and ultimately maintain that weight loss. Just don't expect to see results on your scale tomorrow. A period of time must pass before you will see any measurable weight loss. If you're building a business, you know that you don't start at the level of success you eventually want to reach. It may take years of effort to accomplish this.

Understand the need to be patient. If you become frustrated, you may have forgotten that the end result doesn't occur in an instant. Work must be put forth over a prolonged period of time. Some things may take weeks to accomplish, others may take months and still others, years. You should still enjoy the journey that you take to achieve your desires.

Keep reminding yourself of the difference between instant gratification and delayed gratification. The difference is in how soon personal fulfillment results. By knowing this, you'll have a more realistic understanding of the time commitment involved.

Patience requires a high level of personal insight. Apply this to all aspects of your life. You have to appreciate the fact that there is a master game plan. Maintain a level head and don't panic because you feel things aren't progressing fast enough. Learn to be patient and you will go far feeling and looking great.

49.

Bring Your Manners With You Everywhere You Go

Good manners should be a part of your life at all times. They're not meant to be used only for the purpose of getting something, so don't discard them once you get what you want. Civility is easily lost unless you work at maintaining it. Good manners can be contagious. If you are well mannered, others will be impressed in the way you handle yourself and will want to emulate your actions.

Showing good manners should be a way of life. Incorporate them into your daily activities. At work it would be hypocritical to be well-mannered when dealing with a customer on the phone and then to be rude to the people you work with when you get off the phone. Everyone you encounter should be treated with the same courtesy. Be consistent in your interactions with others and they will appreciate it.

Don't use good manners for only a self-serving purpose or in an evil or manipulative way. Once you get what you want, don't forget your manners. You've probably been in situations where proper manners got you something you desired, but that shouldn't be the main reason for using them. Good manners should have a positive effect on the people with whom you interact.

Work at maintaining your manners. You'll find it easy to be courteous in certain situations where being mannerly is the rule rather than the exception. It may be more difficult to be polite in other situations. The tougher situations will challenge you to maintain your civility, so be strong when you tread in those waters.

If you conduct yourself in the best way possible when you're around others, they may want to follow in your footsteps. People who are well mannered appear to be in better control of their lives. They seem more confident and intelligent. They also seem to have a lot going for them. If you have good manners, that's exactly how you will appear to others.

50.

Learn How To Gain The Emotional Benefits Of A Vacation Without Actually Going On One

Any time people feel overworked or overwhelmed in their lives they tell themselves that they need a vacation. What they basically want is an escape from the daily grind. They want to step away from the hassles of life so they can have time for themselves and their families. People want to have some fun and go places they find exciting and fascinating. Before they leave for vacation, they've already gained an emotional lift because of the excitement they feel anticipating their trip.

Once on vacation, all sorts of pleasant emotions start to take over. People feel like they're back in a carefree environment, very much like they once felt during summer vacation from school. When people return from vacation, however, they immediately start to worry about all the issues they left unresolved at work or at home. After they return to work, they almost feel like they've never gone on vacation. All of their positive emotions seem to have disappeared. These feelings have to do with people's perspectives on their lives. If they feel bad about working but feel good about vacations, it's because they're telling themselves to feel that way.

Next time be conscious of how you act at work the week before you go on vacation. You'll probably notice that you aren't getting upset as you usually do. When you leave for vacation, you may actually feel like you're going to miss some of the daily challenges at work. You may notice yourself acting differently and treating others around you better. You may be in a lighter mood and feel better about work simply because you know you're heading off on a vacation.

Why should you have a positive attitude about work only when you're ready to go on vacation? For that matter, why should you have a positive attitude in general only when you're on vacation? If these are the only times in your life that you are feeling like yourself, then you must go around with a negative attitude the rest of the time. Don't allow this to happen. You know that you're capable of being positive in situations other than vacation. You've already learned this because you feel filled with positive emotions the week before you leave for vacation. Try to take the emotions you experience on vacation and apply them to your daily life.

You don't want to feel good about life only when you're away from your home and work environment. Think about why a vacation makes you feel so good. Is the positive feeling because you can spend so much more time with your family? If so, try to adjust your life so you can be with your family more when you're not on vacation. Is the positive feeling you get before vacation caused by the excitement of having something fun planned in your life? If so, plan to do more fun things after work and on the weekends, not just while on vacation.

When you're coming home from vacation, do you start to dread all the things awaiting you at work? If so, simply practice the technique of putting negative thoughts out of your head. Vacation fills you with pleasant emotions that you can capture and apply in your daily life. You will feel great doing this.

51.

Try Not To Push The Panic Button

Is there something that makes you panic? Does it make you stop cold in your tracks? Recognize it when it happens and do what's necessary to decrease your level of panic.

Resolve future panic episodes by being mentally prepared for a multitude of scenarios that could occur in any given situation. Once you do this, you'll be ready to face a challenge. You just need to think out what could happen ahead of time and know what to do in each case. Instead of pushing a panic button, have a plan of action ready. NASA sends people into outer space but doesn't have a giant panic button to push when obstacles spring up. Instead, NASA tells everyone to remain calm and work on the problem. Apply this principle to your life and you'll feel better because of it.

Does an exam make you panic? Do you panic when you try to get everyone out of the house in the morning? Do you want to panic when you have to learn something new related to work? Does meeting new people create a level of panic? Does trying to get through the work day create this? When you feel that way, you want to be anywhere but where you are. Learn to understand the position in which you've just been put. For things that you panic over, maximize your state of readiness. It will help you minimize the future apprehension.

Practice what you'd do in a certain situation and think over what the possible outcomes could be. Tell yourself if outcome A occurs you'll do the following. However, if outcome B occurs, then you will do something different. Think through as many scenarios as you can and come up with appropriate actions to take. By taking this approach to what panics you, you'll soon see that you can remain in control.

Situations that you used to dread will now become fun for you because they'll be more like a game. Your attitude will improve your chances of success. You'll impress yourself by correctly anticipating events before they even happen. It's so neat that you'll think to yourself, "How can anything get easier? I can't believe I used to panic over this!"

Whenever you get into a position where you panic, ask yourself if this is what NASA would do. NASA simulates potential problems with their astronauts before they ever leave the ground. Astronauts spend more time on earth training for their mission than they do in actual space flight. They rehearse situations that may never happen because doing so makes the astronauts more confident of themselves and their abilities. They realize a new problem is just something to be worked out. Although being an astronaut is one of the more stressful careers anyone could have, astronauts give the impression that panic is never an issue for them.

Try not to push the panic button. You have a good idea how to go about doing this and you'll get better at it the more you practice. Soon you'll have a new outlook on the challenging situation. You'll find yourself feeling great.

52.

Endure The Rough Times Because You Will Get Through Them

Some people have faced huge obstacles and suffered great hardships in their lives. You've heard stories of how they survived and became stronger, regardless of what confronted them. Because these people have the will to endure, they were soon over the rough times and able to get on with their lives.

When you are confronted with extreme difficulties, take care of yourself. Protect your health and well-being at these moments. Be the proud person that you are and continue to do what's good for you. Don't forget everything you've learned. As you work through the rough times, make sure you're not doing anything that will hurt you. When these periods subside, your pride in yourself will be even stronger than before. You'll feel as if you canoed down the Colorado River rapids not knowing if you could ever get through it. At the end of the rapids, you see smooth water ahead and when you reach it, you realize you have survived.

Enduring the rough times will make you feel great. During these periods in your life, keep in mind that there's always hope and that with hope comes a feeling of calmness. Your optimism will carry you through. Continue to feel good about yourself at these times and you'll feel great to have gotten through it.

53.

Seek Out Athletic Competition

With athletic competition you can experience the highest highs and the lowest lows that professional athletes do. When you compete, it's the emotions of the game that are the lasting memories. Experiencing these emotions is what keeps you coming back for more. You don't have to be the best at the game to gain this benefit. You can be a weekend player or a once-a-month player. You can compete in a very social way, perhaps with a partner against other couples. You don't have to see your opponent bleed in order to feel you competed successfully.

You probably first felt the thrill of competing in a game when you were in grade school. If you were on your school team or involved in an intramural sport, you'll remember the excitement of getting ready to play on game day. You thought about how you would play and if you were going to win or lose. You were excited because you were playing in a real game and not another practice. You looked forward to putting on your uniform and thought it was the greatest thing. You also thought about who was going to come to watch you play. After the game you would get together with your friends and talk about the great plays and how much fun it was. You may have found moments during the game you thought were funny and you'd laugh out loud after the game when you recreated those moments with your friends or family. The joys of the game and competition were not only felt while the game was being played, but were experienced both before and after the game.

Remember how you would look forward to the next game. You would think about it every day and talk about how you couldn't wait to play again. If you had the opportunity to continue to compete in athletics when you were in high school, college or beyond, you'll remember how the thrill was still there. After you leave formal school surroundings it may take more of an effort to find these activities.

You may have to go to your local park to get involved with baseball, basketball or soccer; or to an athletic club to find tennis or racketball; or you may need to find a local club which sponsors and organizes the sport you want to play. The thrill and excitement you'll experience from competing now is no different from what you experienced in grade school. If you hit a game winning home run or scored a game winning goal back in seventh grade, you know that if you repeat that twenty years later, it felt just as good.

If you're not a professional athlete competing in your sport, realize that you're competing in a social way. You have to be realistic about what level you can compete at. Begin with a level that's right for your age and ability. You don't want to hurt yourself because you did too much too soon. You would then have to recover which would cause you to miss playing while you recovered. Get started at the right speed and level for your needs and progress from there.

Regain the fun and excitement you felt as a child. Play a sport that gives you the opportunity to compete against others. Win or lose, you'll gain due to the benefits athletic competition provides. It will make you feel great and it's a wonderful way to stay active.

54.

Concentrate On What You Can Do, Not On What You Cannot Do

Know your strengths and weaknesses. Know what you like to do and what you don't like to do. Don't spend all your time on things which will get you nowhere. Try to concentrate more on those things you can do well and get busy doing them. If you spend a majority of your time on things you can do and less time on things you cannot do, you'll become much more productive.

Think about a project you started around the house or something you tried to fix. Did you have any understanding of how to go about doing it? Did you not bother to seek out information on how to fix it but just went ahead and tried to fix it anyway? If you did it that way, you know how long it took you to get nowhere. You may have ruined what you tried to fix. You may have made the problem worse than it was before you started. Consider this an example of what not to do.

Will you commit some time to learn what needs to be done when you don't really know how to do something? If not, get someone who does know what to do to take care of the problem. People who have professional careers in business have sustained bad leg injuries when they fell off the roofs of their homes trying to fix or paint something high up. Others have injured themselves severely trying to fix broken garage doors. When these people injure themselves, they aren't able to do their own job for many months. Avoid hurting yourself or someone else as a result of attempting something you shouldn't be doing.

The best situation is to be able to spend more time on things you enjoy and can do effectively. You may not understand why you're having so much fun at work or on a project until you realize that you're doing something you are good at and enjoy. You'll waste less time when you're in this mode. You will feel great when you start to concentrate on what you can do and not what you cannot do.

55.

Watch A Sporting Event And Act Like A True Fan Of The Game

It's time to let yourself loose and watch a live sporting event. It's nothing like a television rerun. Be prepared to become completely engrossed in watching something for pure enjoyment. Root for your team; it's time to get emotional. Express yourself; it's time to be vocal. No matter what the outcome of the game, realize that it's not a life or death type of thing. Everyone will be around after it's over. Life will go on. You'll feel great becoming immersed in the excitement.

A live sporting event is what you need. The exciting thing is the event is happening live, so you don't know what will happen. You're on edge with anticipation. One minute the team is doing great and the next minute it looks like the team is getting murdered. Your emotions are pulled in ever way possible. A basketball game or hockey game has fast action and is exciting. A close scoring baseball game or soccer game can also have your emotions running high. Pick the sport and team that you can get into and enjoy following. The team you pick doesn't have to be from your area; it may be many states away. If you can watch the sporting event in person this is very exciting. You can be energized by all the others around you. But watching on a big screen television at a bar or at home can be just as meaningful.

Getting involved in a live sporting event is completely different than watching a television rerun. In a rerun you already know what the characters will say and what the outcome will be. You can't experience the complete exhilaration you do when live events occur. Watching a television rerun is the same as watching a sports rerun. Once the outcome is known, everything between the beginning and the end doesn't have as much emotional impact on you. Think of how unexciting it is to watch a sporting event rerun in which you first know what the final score was, what the scores were at each quarter and who scored the points.

Become completely engrossed in watching a sporting event. All of your personal troubles and worries will disappear. You'll be mentally freed and able to concentrate instead on something whose sole purpose is to provide you with viewing pleasure. Your own day will seem like a distant memory because what's happening in the game will become the only reality that exists.

Scream and cheer for your team when something great happens. It feels good to root your heart out, so let your emotions lose! It's fun to yell at your team to get them going even if you are sitting at home watching on television. If you feel completely exhausted after the game is over, you'll know you really got into it.

It is always more fun if your team wins but the great thing about watching a sporting event is that you don't have to be personally affected if your team loses. You won't be required to run more wind sprints the entire next week at practice. You won't have to confront the media and explain to them why you played so poorly. No one is going to trade you or demote you from first string to second or third string. You can put the loss out of your mind until the next time you watch the game. You have gained all the emotional benefits of playing without having to suffer any consequences. Immersing yourself in a live sporting event will make you feel great.

56.

Drink Plenty Of Fluid Each Day

Your body loses fluid when you sweat, when you breathe out and when you go to the bathroom. Fluid evaporates from your skin even if you don't see yourself sweating. The activities you do, what you eat and any alcohol you consume will influence how you will lose fluid from your system. Exercising and drinking alcohol will cause you to lose more fluid. Drink plenty of water each day, at least four to five large glasses, to maximize your health.

People who become dehydrated experience actual symptoms of having too little fluid in their systems. They can feel tired, dizzy, crampy and generally ill at ease. If you go from lying down to a standing position quickly and momentarily feel dizzy, you may be suffering from dehydration. Dehydration causes you to have too little fluid in your blood stream. Because of this, when you stand up, an inadequate amount of blood is pumped to your brain. There can be other reasons for dizziness but this is a common one. Fluids are so important to your system that you won't survive if you withhold all fluid from yourself over a period of many days. This discussion of fluids concerns only water, although sports drinks are also very useful. However, if you have a medical condition in which you need to watch and minimize your sodium or sugar intake, you may not want to replenish your lost fluids with sports drinks because they contain sodium and sugar. In these situations, use water instead.

During a typical day when you aren't exercising or actively losing fluid, you should have a minimum of four to five large glasses of water. If you eat three meals a day, and not everyone does, you could have one large glass of water at each meal. When you're exercising, you'll need at least one or two more large glasses of water in addition to your regular intake. Drinking water at breaks during your sporting activities or workouts will help. Football players who practice twice a day in the hot summer can lose five pounds or more during each session. They must replenish this lost fluid before they start the next practice or they may become ill that same day because of dehydration.

You can monitor your own level of hydration. The color of your urine and how often you urinate can aid in determining if you are drinking enough water. When you on the dehydrated side, your urine becomes concentrated and can be very dark yellow in color. You'll also notice that you're not urinating as often as you usually do. When you're well hydrated and have plenty of water in your system, your urine will not look concentrated and will appear more clear than yellow in color. You will also be urinating more times during the day when you're well hydrated. If you have normal kidney function, you should be able to urinate out the excess fluid you take in. If you have concerns about urinating either too little or too frequently each day, see your family physician. You may have a medical condition that's affecting you.

You may notice that you need to urinate after lying flat on your back for awhile. This is caused by increased blood return from the legs back to your heart. There is more blood return from your legs when you are lying flat than when you're standing and the extra blood goes through your heart and then it ultimately passes through your kidneys. Since there is more blood passing through the kidneys, they will produce more urine.

Drinking alcohol can lead to dehydration. You lose more fluid when you drink alcohol because alcohol causes your kidneys to excrete more water. Your body ends up losing more water than it is taking on. When you consume too much alcohol, the resulting dehydration is one reason you experience a hangover and feel awful. The toxic effect of the alcohol is another reason.

You now know a simple way to monitor yourself to determine if you're drinking enough water. You know that being dehydrated can make you feel ill and that drinking alcohol can make you dehydrated. On the other hand, while drinking plenty of water is very healthy, you still don't want to overdo it. If you have concerns about urinating too infrequently or too often, see your family doctor. You'll feel great and maintain your health when you drink the right amount of water each day.

57.

If You Drink Alcohol, Drink Responsibly And In Moderation

People have consumed alcohol for thousands of years. Although they may speak of the pleasure that has been derived from drinking, you know from stories and personal experience that bad things can come from it. If you drink alcohol, drink in moderation and be responsible to yourself and others for your actions.

Wait until you're of legal age before you drink alcohol. There are teenagers who are already alcoholics before they set foot on a college campus. It's even more unfortunate that some children are alcoholics before they start high school. Encourage others to wait until the legal age to drink because it will decrease their chances of suffering long term alcohol abuse. If they have to find other means of entertaining themselves during their formative years, they won't grow up thinking that they always need to be drunk in order to feel comfortable enough to talk to others, have fun or get through life. If they wait to start drinking until they reach the legal age, they'll be more responsible for their actions because they should be mature enough by then to put their drinking into the proper perspective. Obviously, even people who wait to start drinking may not act maturely and can suffer from alcohol abuse. However, people who start to drink earlier and heavily are at even greater risk. It's important for pregnant women not to drink alcohol due to the risk to the baby.

Alcohol certainly has its negative points. Drinking in excess may make you irrational or cause you to say hurtful things to those you love. It may make you unable to drive your car properly, resulting in a serious accident and injury to yourself or others. It may leave you with a terrible hangover or feeling violently ill because of it. Don't forget that it will also leave you dehydrated. Bad events can happen from alcohol abuse.

Now that the negative things have been discussed, some good things can also be said about alcohol. The key to alcohol's positive side is in drinking alcohol responsibly and in moderation. Drinking a glass of red wine a day can provide health benefits. But remember, this means having one glass of red wine a day and not eight glasses of wine within several hours. By drinking red wine in moderation, you can actually benefit yourself. Speak to your family doctor about it. If you don't really like red wine, don't start drinking it because you can find other ways to maximize your health.

The initial effect of drinking alcohol in moderation is that it may make a person feel more lively, even though alcohol is a depressant. What alcohol first does is suppress your inhibition. For example, you might find it easier to start talking to others after a drink. If you drink too much, it will continue to suppress you until you pass out.

By being responsible for drinking alcohol, you won't put yourself and others in harm's way. Don't let your emotions reach to the point where you say offensive things to others and become violent. You must be responsible enough not to drive if you're intoxicated. Wait for several hours after you have stopped drinking before attempting to drive, or have a designated driver available. When you do get in the car, whether you're driving or not, wear your seat belt and make sure the other people are wearing theirs. If you drink alcohol, drink responsibly and in moderation.

58.

Say No To Drugs

If you are now doing illegal drugs, stop! If you are considering doing illegal drugs in the future, don't do it! Doing drugs will cause great mental anguish but also significant physical problems. People die early deaths when their hearts and lungs stop working because of illegal drugs. There will be nothing to be gained and everything to lose if you take the path of illegal drug use. If you have prescription medication or over the counter medication that you need to take don't abuse it. If you have acquaintances who do drugs, don't allow them to pressure you or embarrass you into doing drugs with them. They may tell you that you aren't a friend of theirs if you won't participate with them. You need to tell them that they must not be friends of yours if they're trying to get you to do something that will hurt you. Get them help.

Drugs that are prescribed to you by a physician must be treated with respect. If you're taking prescription pain medicine, tranquilizers or stimulants, you must not self abuse your medicine or share it with other people. You can do great harm to yourself or to the people with whom you share. Even your physician may not realize you're using medication improperly. If your health is suffering because you're overmedicating yourself, you must inform your physician. You'll only suffer if you don't get help.

Don't abuse over the counter medicine. Over the counter medication is medication that you can buy right off the store's shelves without a prescription. Even this type of medicine has the potential to be abused. Many drugs that once were available only by prescription have now become available over the counter. Don't be fooled into thinking that this type of medication is not strong because it can definitely lead to problems if not used properly.

Some types of illegal drugs, like heroin, are injected directly into a vein. Along with the effects of the drug itself, illegal drug users also hurt themselves physically at the injection sites they use. Illegal injectable drugs are usually bought as a powder and then heated to allow it to melt. Once in liquid form, it is injected into a vein. These drugs generally have a talc type power associated with them. When the drug is injected the talc especially, irritates the vein which can then become infected. Ultimately, the vein will clot off from repeated injections. A new vein must be found but eventually all the accessible veins are used up. Other sites of injection are then found. The undersurface of the tongue has large veins which are injected. Veins of the face and neck are used. Once drug addicts can find no more veins, they start doing something called "skin popping", which means they inject the drug under the skin into the fat. The drug is then absorbed into the system.

Heroin addicts use the vein route first because the rush is so quick and intense. They don't like to skin pop because the rush takes longer and is less powerful. Skin popping can cause the skin to become infected and ulcerated. It's a very ugly site and drug addicts keep their arms and legs covered to hide the non-healing open sores.

Snorting cocaine into the nose is equally bad. When snorted, cocaine is absorbed into the system through the red lining inside the nose called the mucosa. Repeated abuse by snorting cocaine will lead to massive nose bleeds. It can kill the cartilage that holds the nose up and cause it to look flattened and scooped out, like a punched out boxer's nose.

Get help for people who have taken the unfortunate course of drug abuse. Say no to illegal drugs. Respect the prescription medication you are given. Respect over the counter medication. You will feel and look great because of it.

59.

Take A Multivitamin And Mineral Supplement

Vitamins and minerals are responsible for allowing our bodies to function properly, which allows us to maintain our health. Eating a well balanced diet is the best way for a healthy person to get these vitamins and minerals. If you find that you're having difficulty eating a well-balanced diet, you can take a multivitamin and mineral supplement. Even if you think you eat well, you still may not be getting all the important vitamins and minerals in sufficient amounts.

To supplement your dietary intake, take a single multivitamin and mineral supplement tablet once a day. A multivitamin tablet may have less than 100 mg of vitamin C in it but this is still above an adult's recommended dietary allowance (RDA), as established by health experts. Additionally, you can take a vitamin C supplement of 500 mg (milligrams) to 1000 mg once a day. This higher dose is well above the daily RDA but is still considered safe provided a person is healthy. Speak to your doctor about this and adding or increasing any other supplements or antioxidants like vitamin E. You can find multivitamins and mineral supplements at grocery stores, nutrition stores and your local pharmacy. The RDA listing will be on the bottle.

Children, pregnant women, women trying get pregnant and women who are breast feeding are special groups who must take the correct dosage of vitamins for their special needs. There are specific children's multivitamins and prenatal vitamins already available that are formulated differently than typical adult vitamins. Always read the label of the vitamin container to make sure that the vitamins are appropriate for your circumstances. On the label you should find the dosage of each substance that is in the pill. You should also find the percentage of the recommended dietary allowance (RDA) it provides. A value of 50 means it provides 50% of the daily recommended needs. A value of 100 means it provides 100% of the daily recommended needs. A value of 200 means it provides 200%, and so on.

Vitamins are divided into two large categories, fat soluble and water soluble. The fat soluble vitamins are vitamin K, vitamin E, vitamin A and vitamin D. A simple way to remember this for the rest of your life is to think about a "fat kid". The work "fat" refers to fat soluble vitamins. The work "kid" should be thought of as being spelled "KEAD". Each letter in the word "KEAD" refers to a fat soluble vitamin: vitamin K, vitamin E, vitamin A and vitamin D. To recall the fat soluble vitamins now think of "fat KEAD". It's important to know which vitamins are fat soluble because when you take larger doses it's easier to overdose on them than on water soluble vitamins. An overdose of fat soluble vitamins can lead to toxicity because the excess will be absorbed by your fat cells, stay in your body and not easily be cleared out of your system.

If water soluble vitamins are taken in excess, they will be excreted out of your system through the kidneys, as long as you have normal kidney function. The point to remember is that toxicity to your system may develop more easily with fat soluble vitamins than with water soluble ones. Pay special attention to the dosage of a fat soluble vitamin you may be taking.

Vitamin C and the group of eight separate vitamins known as the B complex vitamins are water soluble. The B complex vitamins are vitamin B-1 (thiamine), vitamin B-2 (riboflavin), niacin, vitamin B-6, vitamin B-12, pantothenic acid, biotin and folic acid. When they were first identified, the B complex vitamins where believed to only be a single vitamin but further study identified the eight different vitamins.

Your body produces five vitamins: vitamin D, vitamin K, biotin, niacin and pantothenic acid. Vitamin K and Biotin will be added to the vitamin supplement but only as a fraction of the daily requirement. Vitamin D, niacin and pantothenic acid can be found in the multivitamin tablet pill at 100% of the recommended dietary allowance.

Each vitamin has a separate function. Vitamin C is important for collagen formation in the skin, wound healing and healthy bones and teeth. In extreme cases vitamin B-1 deficiency can cause heart problems and neuromuscular problems including leg numbness, tingling and muscle weakness. Vitamin B-12 and folic acid are involved in blood formation. Deficiencies of these two vitamins can lead to anemia, which is a decreased blood count. People who are strict vegetarians may be lacking vitamin B-12 because it is naturally found in eggs, fish, liver, meat and poultry. Eat a well-balanced diet in order to get the full range of vitamins. Eating only one type of food source won't give you all the vitamins you need.

Vitamins are found naturally in such substance as leafy green vegetables, fruits, eggs, fish, grain, milk and poultry. Your doctor can check your vitamin and mineral supplements and advise you if you need to add a new supplement or take more of a specific vitamin or mineral than you get from the once a day multivitamin and mineral supplement. For women, your doctor may recommend increasing your dissolvable calcium intake.

To maximize your health, especially if you don't feel you're eating a well-balanced diet, take a multivitamin and mineral supplement. Add a separate vitamin C supplement to this. Add any others which your doctor may advise, like the antioxidant, vitamin E. Vitamin C also is an antioxidant. The specific pill you take is dependant on your age, state of health and for women, whether there is a pregnancy, soon to be pregnancy or active breast feeding. Make sure you recognize the proper category you fall into. The dosing of vitamins and minerals and what vitamins are included or excluded is dependant on this.

60.

Minimize Your Exposure To Catching A Cold And The Flu

Estimate the number of days you've stayed home from work each year when you came down with a cold or the flu. Even if you've just grinned and bared your illness and went to work, you probably remember how bad you felt for a period of time. You may still have felt run down for weeks after you recovered. Maybe you missed fun activities or even a planned vacation because of your illness. It's never convenient to get a cold or the flu. Take the necessary precautions and minimize your exposure.

The common cold and the flu are caused by viruses. You can reduce the majority of colds and flu you catch if you take precautions. Staying away from a person who is ill is one of them. In many cases you are exposed to a virus when you touch an object which has the virus on it or you come in contact with someone who has the virus. Once your hand comes in contact with the virus, without realizing it, you then touch or scratch your nose or mouth. You have just inoculated yourself with the virus. Most of these illnesses occur because you come in contact with the virus and unnecessarily expose yourself to it.

Plan to reduce your exposure. During the cold and flu season, stop yourself from touching your nose or mouth after you shake someone's hand. Many people have a habit of doing this. If you observe two people meeting and shaking hands, watch to see how long it takes for one of them to rub their own nose with the hand that was shaken. This person has just inoculated himself with a cold virus if the other person was sick. If you shook hands and now have another person's cold virus on your hand, washing your hands will disinfect them. It will prevent you from inoculating yourself if you later touch your nose or mouth.

When someone coughs or sneezes in your face this can also infect you with a virus. Wash your face and hands immediately if this happens. What if someone has just coughed or sneezed on an object like a book and you didn't see it happen? That's another way to become infected. You won't know the book has been inoculated with a virus. If you pick up the book, you won't realize you have the cold virus on your hand. Once you touch your nose, you'll spread the virus to your respiratory tract without knowing it.

If you're in a large gathering and are shaking many people's hands, keep your hands away from your face. If you're going to eat later, wash your hands to eliminate any virus from them. Do this before you touch food with your hands and put food in your mouth. If you're shaking hands but also munching on appetizers, use a fork or appetizer toothpick to pick up the food. Don't use your bare hands. You can still continue to have manners when meeting others but you can reduce your exposure to viruses that cause colds and flu.

Yearly flu shots are also available. The flu shot will help your immune system fight the virus once you are exposed to it. Not every virus you're exposed to will be covered by the flu shot but a lot of viruses are. Talk to your family doctor to decide if you are a candidate for a flu shot. Finally, remember that washing your hands with soap and water is a simple but highly effective way to protect yourself and others. The best thing to do is still take precautions and minimize your exposure to catching a cold and the flu. If you do catch the flu, your doctor may be able to prescribe you Tamiflu. It may help if you start within 2 days of your flu symptoms.

61.

Protect Your Skin From The Sun

Your skin is the largest organ of your body. Excess exposure to the sun can damage your skin. The sun's ultraviolet rays are the harmful rays and can cause more than a common sunburn. They can lead to premature wrinkling and aging of the skin, precancerous skin changes and skin cancer. Effective ways to protect your skin from the sun's harmful effects include wearing suntan lotion to reduce the ultraviolet rays and wearing protective clothing like a hat, long sleeved shirt and long pants. Seeking out shade under a tree or a sun umbrella is another way to reduce the sun exposure. If you need to get out of the sun completely, go indoors.

The more fair skinned you are, the more you will be affected by the sun's harmful ultraviolet rays. Melanin, which is located in the skin, provides natural protection from sun burning. Since fair skinned individuals have less melanin or skin pigment they have less natural protection from the sun. Darker skinned individuals have greater amounts of melanin and, therefore, greater protection. The amount of melanin or pigment produced by the skin is a major factor in determining what a person's skin tone will be.

Do you have light colored skin, sunburn easily and don't suntan? If so, you're at the greatest risk of sun damage of any skin type. However, even people with other skin types must protect themselves from the sun, because the ultraviolet rays can harm them too and cause sunburn, premature skin wrinkling, precancerous skin changes and skin cancer. Regardless of your skin type, you must protect yourself from the sun and never sunburn.

Wear suntan lotion with a sun protective factor (SPF) of at least 45 or greater. Stores that sell suntan lotion will also carry SPFs that go higher than 45. Buy the highest number available and wear suntan lotion which has both UVA ray and UVB ray protection. The SPF number refers to the protection from the UVB rays. Ultraviolet light is broken down into A, B and C types. UVA refers to ultraviolet light in the A range; UVB refers to ultraviolet light in the B range. UVB rays are the most harmful of these three types. They're responsible for sunburns, premature wrinkling and the degeneration of normal skin to skin cancer. UVA rays lead to tanning of the skin by stimulating the production of melanin. They can enhance the harmful effects that occur because of the UVB rays. UVA rays have been found to cause skin cancer in mice but to a much lesser degree than UVB rays do. Because of the filtering effect of the ozone layer, UVC rays are almost nonexistent on the earth's surface, so they are not a factor in sun protection.

Suntan lotion protects the skin by absorbing harmful rays. The other major type of topical sunscreen works primarily by reflecting the harmful rays away. For example, many life guards on the beach wear zinc oxide on their nose. It's a white cream that's a reflective sunscreen. Although reflective sunscreens like zinc oxide actually provide more protection than suntan lotion which work by absorbing the rays, they are not used as frequently. Because suntan lotions can blend into the skin, they are cosmetically more acceptable to many people.

Wearing protective clothing is another way to minimize your exposure to the sun's harmful rays. When you want to adequately protect your skin, remember that's one of the reasons people in Saudi Arabia completely cover themselves with their garments. The tighter the weave of the material, the less sun gets through. A loosely knit fabric may still allow 30% of the harmful rays through to your skin.

What if you seek shade under an umbrella or tree? That will help, but on a sunny day it won't completely reduce your risk of sunburn. An umbrella top may be loosely woven, allowing some light through. With light reflected off the ground and off the water if you're at a pool or beach, you may only be blocking the rays by 50%. Even in shade, you want to wear suntan lotion, and if needed, protective clothing. Going indoors is the best way to know that you've completely eliminated your risk of sunburn and the other harmful effects.

The sun is warm and energizing. It can lift your spirits and make you feel good. It's fun to go outside on a beautiful, sunny day. For all the good the sun does, it can also do harm. Take adequate precautions to protect yourself from the harmful effects of the sun.

Think Of Wearing Suntan Lotion Before You Go Out In The Sun Like You Think Of Wearing A Seat Belt Before You Drive In A Car

When you get into a car, please don't start driving until you've fastened your seat belt. Hopefully, you realize how important a seat belt is to your safety and the safety of others. Make sure everyone in the car is wearing their seat belt. Be responsible in this way even if you aren't the driver. You definitely understand the importance and safety of a seat belt and you've conditioned yourself to always remember to wear a seat belt every time you get back into a car. You want what's best for you. Think along these same lines when it comes to getting accustomed to wearing suntan lotion. When you go out on a sunny day, have your suntan lotion already applied and have other appropriate protection from the sun with you. You want to condition yourself to always consciously think about protecting your skin before you go out in the sun.

If you are more fair skinned, try to recall a vacation during which you didn't protect yourself from the sun. You may have seriously burned your skin by the second or third day of the vacation. Remember how much pain you were in hours later, when the sunburn became obvious. You probably had to stay in your hotel room for the next several days because any exposure to the sun was too painful for you to tolerate. If you burned your back or chest, think about how difficult it was to lie down comfortably directly on the burned areas. You ruined the rest of your vacation by not initially taking the proper precautions regarding skin care. When you returned home, your skin flaked off for the next two weeks and you needed to vacuum your bed and floor to get rid of all you had shed.

You may remember fair skinned friends who went to an outdoor concert on a hot, sunny day in July or August. Think about the red lobster color they'd turned when you saw them the next day. It may have taken weeks for them to recover from their sunburns.

Recall these stories and others to reinforce your need to protect your skin from the sun. Not only can you prevent the acute damage from a sunburn: pain, redness and skin blistering, but you can minimize effects like premature skin wrinkling, precancerous changes of the skin and sun induced skin cancer.

If you're out in the sun on vacation in places like Florida or Hawaii or outside your home during the summer, you should apply a suntan lotion with a SPF (sun protective factor) of at least 45 or greater. The SPF number tells you how much protection you get from the UVB rays. Get suntan lotion which also has UVA protection. Make sure you get waterproof (water resistant is a more accurate term) lotion, although even then you should reapply the sunblock every hour if you are out swimming. To more accurately describe the suntan lotion products the FDA will require the manufacturers to label the product as a "sunscreen" instead of a "sunblock" and as "water resistant" instead of "waterproof". If you're not swimming, you'll need to reapply the lotion every two to three hours, especially if you're sweating. If you've applied the suntan lotion correctly and frequently enough, you'll find that after a week's vacation swimming out in the sun, you won't be sunburned and your skin will not be in pain or flaking off to any significant degree. You'll be very impressed by how much better you feel when you use suntan lotion. You'll still suntan if you use suntan lotion but you won't need to sunburn first. The suntan will appear days after your first exposure. Although it won't be as intense as if you used no lotion, you'll be much better off in the short and long run.

In the future you'll notice that the SPF number you can buy keeps getting higher and higher. If you can buy suntan lotion with these higher numbers, do so. Lotion with an SPF of 15 will block out approximately 91% of the UVB rays. A suntan lotion with a

SPF of 45 will block up to 95% of the UVB rays. SPF numbers will continue to go higher until lotions someday reach toward 100% UVB blockage.

Think about wearing suntan lotion and protecting your skin from the sun before you even walk out of the house. Consider it as important as you consider wearing a seat belt before you start to drive your car. You will be glad you did this not only because you prevented yourself from burning but because of the benefit you'll derive over the long term.

63.

Who Should Protect Their Skin From The Sun? Children, Adults And Grandparents!

Teach children the importance of protecting their skin from the sun's harmful ultraviolet rays. Make sure they protect their skin by wearing suntan lotion and protective clothing. Have them apply suntan lotion before they go out on a sunny day to play or go swimming. Have suntan lotion easily accessible in the house and also put it in their beach bag so it's always with them. Children need to learn to continue to do this all through their adulthood. It's necessary to protect your skin from the sun at any age. All of the recommendations for sun protection apply equally to children, adults and grandparents.

Children will be grateful to you for showing them how to decrease their episodes of sunburn. They may be too young to appreciate the fact that they'll also decrease the sun induced wrinkling of their skin and the potential for sun induced skin damage and skin cancers, but explain it to them anyway. As they get older, they'll see and appreciate the long term benefits they've received by learning at an early age how to protect their skin from the sun. Think about the dry and wrinkled appearance of the face of a person who's always been out in the sun. They didn't take any steps to minimize the harmful sun effects. You don't want this to happen to you.

As an adult, and even if you are a grandparent, it's still not too late to get started with proper skin protection from the sun. What if you plan to go out in the sun for the next decade and not provide any protection? Your skin would be in a lot worse shape ten years from now then if you protected your skin. Protect your skin to enjoy the benefits later.

The need for sun protection is obvious in the summer time and on warm vacations. Even on cloudy days during the summer up to 80% of the harmful sunrays can still reach you. You can get sunburned on a cloudy day if you don't have on suntan lotion. Sunburns can happen during the fall and spring months too. Depending on how long you're outside, you may need to continue applying suntan lotion. If you go skiing on a winter vacation, you need to wear suntan lotion. It's easy to get a sunburn because the snow reflects a lot of light on your face. The harmful ultraviolet sun rays are less filtered the higher up in altitude you go. It's important to continue to protect your skin in the winter months.

Who should wear at least a SPF 45 suntan lotion along with UVA protection? Everyone should. Regardless of your age, you should purchase the highest SPF you can. The SPF number will be clearly marked on the suntan lotion bottle. If you have a waterproof lotion and you're swimming, reapply the lotion every hour. Children can wear the same suntan lotion that adults do. It's fine to use the same bottle of suntan lotion for the entire family.

Continue this as long as no one develops a skin sensitivity to the lotion. The recommendations for proper sun protection apply to all ages. The younger someone starts using protection the better. No matter what age you are you should continue to protect your skin from the sun.

64.

Do A Self Skin Exam Every Month

Remember that your skin is the largest organ of your body and you want to keep it in the best shape possible. It's important to know what your skin looks like and to do that, you have to exam it. When you examine your skin, you need to look for skin growths that have the potential to develop into skin cancer or are already cancerous.

One type of skin cancer called melanoma actually kills people. The death rate from melanoma is increasing each year because people have a false impression that skin growths don't need to be treated. Half of all the cancer in America are skin cancers. If you wanted to cure half the cancer in America within the next year, you can do it by teaching everyone to do a self skin exam every month and have the suspicious growths treated. See your plastic surgeon about this. It is important to have a professional look at your skin at least once a year because you may still miss identifying skin growths that may need to be treated

It's common for some people to have at least fifty to one hundred abnormal growths already present on their skin. These growths need to be monitored each month. If they change in color, size, shape, become more irregular, become darker, start to bleed, become painful, scab over or act different they should be treated. What if you notice a new growth that has never been present before? If it's still there for over a month or longer, it may need to be treated. Some people can have large skin cancers develop in only a matter of one month.

Many places on your skin can be seen easily but there are other areas that you can't see unless you use a mirror or two sets of mirrors. Use a single mirror to see the front of your scalp, the front of your face, your ears, the front of your neck, your upper chest, your buttock area and the back of your legs. Use two sets of mirrors to see the back of your scalp, behind and inside your ears, the back of your neck and your back.

To determine if your skin is doing fine you need to do a self skin exam once a month. Do this when you get out of the shower since, hopefully, you are naked at this time. Look from the top of your body to the bottoms of your feet. Start by looking in the mirror and look at the front of your scalp, face and neck. Use two mirrors to look at the back of your scalp and neck. If you feel any skin growth on your scalp and you have a thick head of hair, move the hair so you can see what the growth looks like. Also inspect your scalp by moving the hair around and look for any dark, flat or irregular growths.

Next look at the front of your chest, breast and abdomen. Look around your arms and at the palms of your hands and your fingers. Look at your back with two mirrors. Check your groin area and buttocks. Look at the entire circumference of your legs and then at the top of your feet and your toes. You should even check the soles of your feet.

Some skin cancers of the scalp have been first identified by beauticians or hair stylists while cutting their customers' hair. I've diagnosed and treated patients with melanoma and other skin cancers even though they originally came into my office to have breast enlargement procedures or something else done.

During the skin exams I discovered these growths. The other procedures they first came in for were still able to be done but it was fortunate that their skin cancers could also be treated.

Seek out a plastic surgeon to evaluate your skin and teach you the finer points of a self skin exam. Continue to do a self skin exam every month for the rest of your life. What if you do find a growth that has changed in appearance or find a new growth? You can have your plastic surgeon decide if it's appropriate to have the growth removed.

65.

Have Abnormal Skin Growths Removed

What's your next step if you find an abnormal skin growth during your once a month skin examination? Have the abnormal growth evaluated by your family doctor or your plastic surgeon. Your physician can decide if removing the skin growth is the appropriate course of action. Don't think that you have to be older to develop skin cancer. Skin cancers such as melanoma are identified on people who are in their twenties and younger. Basal cell cancer is another type of common skin cancer that's seen in people who are in their mid-thirties. The earlier you have abnormal skin growths treated, the better off you'll be. It's also important to have noncancerous growths removed to prevent them from enlarging and destroying the surrounding skin or growing into skin cancer.

What about the skin cancer called melanoma? It typically starts as a dark, noncancerous growth. The growth continues to change and grow over time until it finally becomes melanoma. Approximately 85% of all melanomas develop this way. It is important to have the skin growths which have the potentially to become cancer removed. By having these growths removed the potential for them to become melanoma is reduced to virtually 0%.

To understand how an abnormal skin growth can vary from being slightly abnormal to significantly abnormal (bordering on skin cancer) think of a room with a ladder in it. The ladder has many rungs and is leaning up against the wall. The ladder reaches to the ceiling of the room. Imagine that this represents a way of thinking about skin. Think of normal skin being at the floor of the room and skin cancer as being at the ceiling or top level.

For your normal skin to become cancer, it has to take a step up each rung of the ladder to ultimately reach the ceiling. With each step up the ladder the skin growth becomes more and more abnormal. The object is to remove abnormal skin growths while they are hopefully still low on the ladder and well away from becoming skin cancer.

Seeing an abnormal skin growth means it is at least on the first rung of the ladder. The abnormal skin growth may be high up on the rungs of the ladder and close to becoming skin cancer. The skin growth may already be skin cancer when you first see it. This would place it at the ceiling position.

Your plastic surgeon will be able to examine an abnormal skin growth and give you an educated guess as to what it is. For an exact diagnosis, the skin growth will be removed and sent to the pathologist for evaluation. In many instances the growth can be removed right in your doctor's office. A medicine is used to numb the skin area before the growth is removed. It may take a week or so to get the final report from the pathologist.

What do you do if you have fifty obvious abnormal growths on your body? Do you remove all of them at the same time? Do they all need to be removed? What should you do in this situation? First, it's important to know if you have a personal or family history of skin cancer. If there is such a history, you need to be aggressive about removing the other skin growths. Second, if you don't have a history of skin cancer but you have had growths removed that where significantly abnormal and bordered on skin cancer, you also want to be aggressive about removing all the growths.

After thoroughly examining your skin growths, your doctor should list the skin growths in order of priority of removal. These growths listed at the top are the ones most suspicious for cancer or are at locations that are significantly deforming the local skin. Growths that are the largest, darkest, most rose, reddened or scaly, most irregular and those that bleed are the most suspicious ones. Many skin cancers, however, will have no symptoms of pain or bleeding associated with them.

With all things being equal, growths on the eyelids, nose, lips, ears, cheeks, neck, scalp, hands and feet need to be treated at a much early stage than the same sized growth on the abdomen. Growths are removed first from areas where there is less skin available to close back together.

As facial growths become larger, they continue to destroy the local surrounding skin and the unique structures of the facial skin. Even if it's not cancerous, a large abnormal skin growth on the face is still destroying local skin. It's best to remove it as early as possible to prevent it from enlarging any further or become cancerous. The cosmetic result will also be better because the smaller they are when they are removed the smaller the scar.

Any skin growths that have been present since your birth are also considered abnormal and should be professionally evaluated. If you are thirty years old and you were born with these skin growths, they've had the opportunity to stay abnormal for over thirty years. That's a long time. Get these growths evaluated by a plastic surgeon and, if recommended, have them removed. Having abnormal skin growths removed will do you great good.

66.

Maximize The Condition Of Your Complexion

There are things you can do today and for the rest of your life to have your skin look as good as possible. Stop eating foods that irritate your skin. To have the best skin possible, stop smoking because smoking cigarettes harms your facial skin. Smoking can also decrease the blood flow to your skin, making it look weathered and aged. Acne should be actively treated to reduce long term scarring. Skin discoloration, dark circles under the eyes and blotchiness, especially in the facial area, should be identified and treated. Look for small blood vessel growths on your face and have something done to make them less visible. Other skin growths of the facial area should be removed.

Some people have had dark circles under their eyes since they were young; others may have gotten them as they grew older. You may have inherited this from your parents. If you are now seeing dark circles under your eyes, do something about it. Once you identify the dark circles, take action!

Cover makeup is the first line of attack against dark circles. Use a makeup that has a powder or paste consistency rather than a liquid. The liquid makeup will streak and be more difficult to apply effectively in this problem area. You can purchase cover makeup containing suntan lotion, an alpha hydroxy acid such as glycolic acid and other agents to improve your skin. The suntan lotion will decrease sunburn, sun induced premature aging and the potential for sun induced skin cancers. Alpha hydroxy acids such as glycolic acid will maximize your skin's smoothness.

Go to the cosmetics counter and have your skin tone properly matched with the makeup. You may have to go to a few places to find the right color match. The cover makeup can be purchased in a lip stick tube. Apply it directly on the skin of both lower eyelids to help conceal the dark circles. Rub it in and feather out the edges with your fingers. In some cases cover makeup will consist of two products. The first product you apply is a base makeup with a purple or green color to it. You then apply a second or final cover makeup on top of the first one. Other treatments for the dark circles may include laser treatment or removal of protruding lower eyelid fat.

When applying makeup, always remember to apply it on both sides of your face at the same anatomic location. If you apply makeup on the left side of the forehead, apply it to the exact opposite site on the right side. This creates normal symmetric facial coloration. If you see someone with a reddened left cheek, this will look abnormal when compared to the right cheek. If both left and right sides of the cheek area are equally reddened as compared to the rest of the face, it will appear more normal.

Generalized skin discoloration and blotchiness can be made less noticeable with cover makeup. This is a great way to immediately have control over your facial skin tone. These conditions may also be helped with topical medications, facial peels or laser treatment.

Small blood vessel growths can be covered with makeup. To eliminate or significantly reduce them, other treatment options are available, such as radiofrequency treatment. This treatment coagulates the blood vessel and stops the blood flow. Laser and injections of medication that cause the blood vessel to scar down and diminish blood flow can be used. Certain blood vessel growths may also be treated by directly excising out the blood vessel.

You want to create the best environment for your skin. Moisturize it to keep it in the best shape. Even with such care, there will always be imperfections on your skin that you want to conceal or eliminate. For those things that can be concealed, a cover makeup is an ideal choice. Even if you've had facial skin rejuvenation procedures, it's still recommended that you continue using cover makeup, sunblock, alpha hydroxy acids and skin moisturizers to maximize your appearance. To eliminate or greatly reduce facial skin blood vessel growths and blotchiness, talk to your plastic surgeon about the most helpful treatments available. Don't wait until any of these conditions have significantly worsened. It's important to start treating your skin early when these conditions are first identified.

67.

Treating Your Skin Well Now Will Have A Direct Impact On How It Will Look Years From Now

There is no delaying what should be done. This is not some thing you want to put on hold. Don't put it on the back burner, take steps to treat your skin well now! The benefits you receive today and for the rest of your life will be tremendous. As the years pass, you'll look back on this day and be grateful you got started when you did. You want the aging process to treat your skin as gently as possible. You don't want the aging process to be more aggressive with you. You don't want to suffer from the sun's harmful effects on your skin for years to come. To avoid things that harm the appearance of your skin, you need to recognize what may be potentially harmful and take action to correct it.

Minimize those things which lead to premature aging and wrinkling of the skin. Minimize situations that injure your skin and lead to the development of sun induced skin damage and sun induced precancerous and cancerous skin growths. Every five to ten years you'll notice changes to your skin that you never thought would happen. But these changes do happen. You want your skin to be in the best shape possible for these future events because if you need plastic surgery to improve the effects of aging, the overall result will be that much better for you.

Keep your skin looking youthful and healthy to reduce the aging effect. If you're in your early thirties, you don't have many wrinkles yet, but you'll be shocked to see all the wrinkles you may have in twenty years. The goal is to minimize potential future changes in your skin. Tremendous benefit can result if you consider you'll be providing your own skin care for the next twenty years.

Imagine if you conducted your own controlled experiment by doing things that are good for your skin on the right side of your face, while doing nothing to take care of the left side.

You can predict what each side of your face would look like. In the future, the right side of your face would have a younger, softer, glowing appearance compared to the older, less healthy appearing left side of your face.

Does it matter what a person's skin looks like in the future? It does! It matters to everyone. In my practice I see people in their mid-seventies who care about how they look and care about the appearance of their skin as those who are in their twenties.

If older patients tell me their appearance isn't really important to them, I tell them that they don't have to feel embarrassed or guilty about caring how they look. I tell them firsthand how everyone cares about their appearance.

The fact is: people are living longer than ever before. This pattern is not changing and may not change in the future. Accept this as a fact. You will care about how your skin looks in the future. Twenty years from now you'll still consider yourself to be young no matter what your age is. Treat your skin well now because it will have a direct impact on how it looks in the future. Your skin is not the same as the roof of a house that needs remodeling. If you want a new roof, you have it completely removed and a new one put in its place. You can't do that with your skin. You have to work with the skin you have, so keep it as youthful and healthy as possibly.

68.

Working Out In The Outdoors Without The Proper Skin Protection Will Harm Your Skin In The Long Term

It feels great to go outside to do your workout. It's good to be surrounded by nature when you're exercising or playing a sport. Days filled with fresh air, sunshine and a clear blue sky are always appreciated. Working out or playing a game is even more exhilarating under these circumstances. When you're exercising or participating in a sport, you know that you're doing a lot of good for yourself by improving your physical appearance and overall physical condition. But getting in great physical shape through outdoor exercise doesn't mean that the appearance of your skin will also benefit. If you're exposing your skin on warm, sunny days and you're not protecting it from the sun's harmful effects, your skin will suffer over the long term.

Even though you're being physical activity, your skin is still subjected to premature aging and wrinkling; drying out; and sun induced skin changes that can lead to skin cancer. People who workout outside and don't protect their skin may appear to be in great physical shape but they don't have healthier appearing skin because the sun is actually damaging it. Make your skin look healthier by protecting it from the sun's harmful ultraviolet rays.

There are people who are avid golfers who have some of the most sun damaged facial skin you can imagine. They may be able to carry their big golf bag around all eighteen holes of the golf course and seem to be in good physical shape because of their activity. However, they have significantly damaged their facial skin. They feel that since they're doing something that's good for their physical well being, it can't do them any harm. The harm comes from not understanding that sun protection is a critical factor and must still be done.

People who run long distances daily outside are also at risk. Though they may be doing their cardiovascular endurance a great service, without sun protection like suntan lotion and protective clothing they're damaging their facial skin and any other skin that's exposed. The dilemma is apparent when you see people who are in great physical shape but they look older than they are because of sun damage to their facial skin. People may not realize that is why they look so wrinkled even though they're physical fit.

If you like to do outside projects like gardening, landscaping and yard work, you're equally at risk. Recall the image of an elderly farmer's face. The dry, weathered, wrinkled skin looks like it's been beaten relentlessly year after year. All the hard years of working outside show on their face. There is no escape from the damage the sun will do to your skin unless you take active measures to protect yourself. Prevent long term damage to your skin. Provide appropriate sun protection when you're outside enjoying your workout or any other activity.

69.

Stop Worrying About Not Getting A Dark Suntan

Getting the intensely dark suntan you've always wanted is not worth it. If it's been achieved by burning your skin for weeks at a time each year it's the wrong thing to do. Whenever you're outside, protect you skin with suntan lotion. You'll still get a tan but the color will probably be lighter than if you hadn't used any lotion. Without proper sun protection, as you reach your thirties, forties and beyond you'll be replacing the youthful appearance and dark tanned skin you had as a teenager with dry, leathery, wrinkled, spotty, unhealthy, aged skin.

Examine your skin at the end of the summer to make a mental note of how much you can tan when you safely expose yourself to the sun. You'll then know the maximum amount of tanning you can achieve when using suntan lotion.

What about tanning booths? Not all tanning booths are alike. Some are much more dangerous than others for long term damage to your skin and it's hard for most people to identify which these are. You don't need to have a tanning booth induced tan before you start your vacation. If you wear suntan lotion and use proper precautions starting your first day of vacation, you can minimize your risk of sunburn.

If you want a darker complexion, an option is to use cover makeup with a darker coloration in it. Try to get a brand with a sunblock and alpha hydroxy acid added. While the makeup is giving you a darker complexion, the sunblock will protect your skin and the alpha hydroxy acid will make it smooth.

Do you have a skin type that never tans? If so, all you may have done in the past is suffer with a sunburn without ever tanning your skin. Relax. Don't try to beat the system. Use a darker makeup if you want to give the illusion of tanned skin. Spray on tanning or self applied tanning products can help. And remember: if you don't tan, it's especially important to protect your skin from the harmful effects of the sun!

There was a time in history when it was in vogue to not have a suntan. During the Middle Ages people who were wealthy did not have to work the fields or tend to the live stock. You can see these pale complexioned people depicted in artwork from that period. Their higher status was demonstrated by how pale they were. The paler their complexions, the less likely it was they did manual outdoor labor.

What if you have the type of skin that tans after a limited amount of protected sun exposure? Be happy! But remember to still protect your skin over the long term. Even though you have a darker complexion without proper sun protection you can still cause your skin to look more aged than you actually are. Stop worrying about not getting a dark suntan and concentrate on protecting your skin from the sun's harmful effects. The rest will take care of itself.

70.

What About The More Exotic Ways To Smooth Skin?

There are many stories of people seeking the fountain of youth. You may have heard you can attain eternal youth by applying a liquid only found in a certain region of the world or by going to a particular fountain or stream and bathing in it. For centuries people have tried a variety of things to improve their skin, including milk baths, mud baths, body wrappings in sea weed and the application of freshly cut apples and other fruits directly on the skin. What is all of this about and how does it apply to modern ways of making yourself look great?

These "fountains of youth" may provide some benefit to the skin, so their use was continued. Although it wasn't apparent why these things worked, the fact that they did show results was enough reason to continue using them. The collective knowledge available in the past did not allow for a scientific explanation. These youth enhancing practices were deliberately shrouded in mystery because the people who had access to their ingredients did not want others to know the secret of their magic potions. They wanted their solutions to appear to have magical powers.

How can bathing in milk do anything to improve your skin? Sour milk has a substance called lactic acid which is an alpha hydroxy acid. Alpha hydroxy acids are not effective against wrinkles, but when applied to the skin, this very type of acid has been found to help soften skin texture by acting as an exfoliant. The skin's rough spots may be lessened and it's general appearance improved. I would not necessarily recommend that someone bathe daily in sour milk but thanks to modern science, today you can apply the active agent (alpha hydroxy acid) to your skin without having to immerse yourself in milk.

What about a mud bath? In the wilds of Africa and South America, applying mud to your skin had a useful purpose. When the mud dried it would protect you from the ravages of the sun. Your skin wouldn't burn while covered with mud, so it was used as a suntan lotion before suntan lotion was ever available in a bottle. A thick layer of mud would also prevent you from getting bitten by small insects. Mud protected your skin not only from the sun but from those pesky nuisances.

Fruits such as apples have been sliced and applied to the eyelids and rest of the face to try and improve the condition of the facial skin. An apple is a natural source for maltic acid. Maltic acid is another example of an alpha hydroxy acid which can exfoliate the skin and smooth it.

Sugar cane is a natural source for glycolic acid. This acid is in the alpha hydroxy acid family and, like the acids in sour milk and apples, it can have a positive affect on your skin by acting as an exfoliant. The alpha hydroxy acid is the active ingredient responsible for its positive effect on your skin and is available to the public. The concentration of the alpha hydroxy acid is much weaker in nature than in commercially available solutions.

Knowing why some of these treatments have been used for such a long time and are still around today is fascinating. If you have the opportunity to indulge in them at a health spa, the more power to you. If you want to get the most benefit from alpha hydroxy acids like glycolic acid, you can buy cover makeup and skin lotions that already contain the glycolic acid solution. You'll be able to apply them to your skin daily. The more exotic ways of smoothing your skin don't seem so exotic once the mystery is removed.

71.

Body Massage

A massage is one of the joys in life. You know it will make you feel better because you'll be more relaxed and less stiff. Previous muscle soreness may be relieved after the massage. A massage can be done to your skin and fat only, primarily to the muscles or all the way down to the bone. Even animals like to get into the act. Your family pet will come up to you and not go away until you start to rub them. Animals will lie down and roll on their back as if they were shot with a tranquilizer dart once you start massaging their bodies. It will be amusing how they give themselves to you.

Have someone give you a massage. They don't have to be a professional. As long as they don't do it hard enough to hurt you it will be safe. Having a massage done by a person trained in massage is great. There will be certain techniques they use that will feel better than other techniques. Take note so you know what they're doing to make it feel so good. Ask them to show you how they use their hands to create such a benefit to your body.

Having certain parts of your body massaged will make you feel more relaxed than others. For some it is the back of the neck, for others the bottom of the feet. Learn which parts of your body this applies to. If you're getting a short massage, ask for the technique which does the best job. Have the most time on the location on your body that is the most rewarding.

What layers of tissue below the skin are being massaged? Immediately below the skin is a layer of fat. Below the fat layer is the muscle. In most areas bone is below the layer of muscle. Depending on the location, there may not be a muscle layer between the fat layer and the bone. For example, the top of your fingers have a tendon which originated from a muscle in the forearm. Deep pressure massage to the top of your fingers will massage skin, fat, tendon of the muscle and bone, but not any muscle.

Massaging certain areas of your body may cause a shooting pain in that area or region. Don't be alarmed by this. The pain is usually caused by a nerve within the tissue being manipulated or stretched. The nerve is reacting to the pressure being applied over it. Your funny bone is an example of this. Recall back in grade school when you had your elbow resting on a stack of books. If the inside of your elbow slide off the books, you felt a tingling and electrical jolt that went from your elbow down to the side of your hand and little finger. This sensation was caused by overstimulating the ulnar nerve, which travels through the inner elbow region and runs to your hand. Even though you stimulated the nerve at the elbow, you still felt symptoms all the way to your finger.

Body massage may help in more ways than only relaxing the specific area that is massaged. Getting a massage is a pure pleasure. If no one is available to give you a massage then give yourself a massage for five or ten minutes. It will make you feel great.

72.

What You See In The Mirror And Want Improved May Be Helped With Plastic Surgery

You no longer have to look in the mirror and think nothing can be done to improve what you see. You live in an era in which your appearance and shape can be improved. You don't have to settle with what fate has dealt you. You can control your appearance and your physical shape and may improve them by having plastic surgery.

It's important to keep yourself and your skin in great condition throughout your life. You want to be in the best shape and have the best skin possible for your age, so do all the right things to keep yourself and your skin as youthful and healthy as possible. If you do this, you'll benefit even more when having plastic surgery. Plastic surgery is not a substitute for a healthy lifestyle but should complement what you are already doing for yourself.

Even though you're doing everything to keep your skin as youthful as possible, as you grow older you'll still see signs of aging. You may notice more skin sagging around the eyes, mouth, jaw line and neck. Your neck may start to look fatter even if you haven't gained any significant amount of weight. Fine wrinkles will start to become more noticeable on your forehead, around the eyes, on your nose, and around your mouth, cheeks and the neck.

Plastic surgery techniques exist which will help give you a more youthful appearance. A question commonly asked is when can someone benefit from these types of treatment? You can receive and benefit from the treatment as soon as you notice signs of aging. The earlier you have the treatment, the greater the benefit you receive. Plastic surgery can help make you more youthful appearing. It can also help maintain the youthful appearance you may already have.

When plastic surgery care is rendered at the first signs of aging, it will help maintain the overall appearance of your youthfulness. Can these treatments be repeated in the future? The answer is yes. To maintain a youthful appearance for as long as possible, undergoing retreatment is a great option. The goal is to have you look as youthful as possible and still have you look like yourself. You want others to see you and think that you must have been on a vacation or are well rested because you look so good.

Poorly shaped noses can be reshaped. Receding chins can be made more prominent. The shape that a woman may acquire as a result of having children can be improved. Women who have lost breast volume and develop drooping breasts following a pregnancy and women who have had small breasts all their lives can have their breasts enlarged. Women with large, pendulous breasts that cause headache in addition to back, neck and shoulder pain can have the breasts lifted and reduced in size. Fat excess of the breast, arms, abdomen, hips, inner thighs, knees and calves can be improved with plastic surgery. Skin and fat excess can be removed and the skin can be tightened. Plastic surgery can also help your appearance in many other ways.

73.

Fine Wrinkles And Blotchiness Of The Face Can Be Improved With Laser Skin Resurfacing

Lasers have been available for medical use since the 1960s. The earliest lasers could only remove a thick layer of skin, which made them unfeasible for the treatment of fine wrinkles. In the early 1990's a carbon dioxide laser was the first laser successfully used to treat fine facial wrinkles. Now technology has progressed to the point where a laser can remove surface skin by only a fraction of a millimeter at a time.

While the carbon dioxide laser is still used for skin resurfacing, other types of laser systems, such as the Erbium laser, are also available. Combinations of laser systems, like an Erbium and carbon dioxide laser, are used as well. Since laser technology progresses not in decades but year to year, just like the computer industry, new laser systems for the treatment of fine wrinkles will continually be coming onto the scene.

Laser skin resurfacing is a marvelous way to treat fine wrinkles of the face. The cheeks, forehead, upper and lower eyelids, crow's feet at the outer corner of the eyes, and fine wrinkles around the bridge of the nose and wrinkles of the upper and lower lip can benefit from laser skin resurfacing. The entire facial skin can be treated at the same time and blotchiness of the facial skin can be improved.

By knowing the anatomy of your skin, you'll understand how laser skin resurfacing works and how your skin heals. The outermost layer of your skin is called the epidermis; the layer below is called the dermis. The epidermis contains cells called melanocytes that make the skin pigment called melanin. Melanin is one very important factor among several that give your skin its color. Melanin production increased when you suntan. The epidermis is the protective covering of the skin. The epidermis is where a lot of the skin blotchiness resides. The shedding of the epidermis' top layer is what gives you flaky skin.

The dermis or bottom layer of your skin makes up about 90% of your skin's total skin thickness. It contains collagen, which gives great strength to your skin. The sweat glands in the dermis are the source of perspiration. The dermis also has hair follicles within it. Each single hair follicle produces a single hair that comes to the surface of your skin through the hair shaft. Sebaceous glands in the dermis open into the hair shaft. These sebaceous glands are responsible for the oiliness of your skin.

Fine facial wrinkles are treated with laser skin resurfacing by removing the entire layer of the epidermis and the upper portion of the dermis. The skin heals because new skin is made from the sweat glands, hair follicle shafts and sebaceous glands contained in the remaining dermis. The edges of the untreated skin also produce new skin at the treatment sites. Once the damaged surface skin is removed, the skin will scab for a period of one to two weeks as it heals. After this a cover makeup can be applied. Previous skin blotchiness will be improved, as might precancerous skin conditions. If someone is taking an acne medication called Accutane, this must be stopped for six months to one year before laser skin resurfacing can be safely done. The procedure can be done under local anesthesia, intravenous sedation, where an I.V. is started and sleep inducing medicine is given to make you sleepy, or under general anesthesia. As with any procedure, complications to watch for include but are not limited to infection, bleeding, scarring and skin color changes. After healing, the skin will have a softer, glowing, healthier, more youthful appearance.

74.

Laser Skin Resurfacing Can Be Repeated In The Future

Laser skin resurfacing should not be thought of as a treatment that can only be done one time and never again. That would be like thinking makeup could only be applied to your face once in your life. After your skin is improved with laser skin resurfacing, it will look more youthful. You'll have to recall what age you were when you remembered your skin looked that good. After the treatment your skin will still undergo the aging process; so some years later you may decide you'd like to have laser skin resurfacing repeated to regain the benefit to your skin.

As the decades march on you'll find it's best to maintain the healthy appearance of your skin. Laser skin resurfacing makes this a reality. Many other things also contribute to maintaining your skin's healthy appearance including, but not limited to, protecting your skin from the sun, using an alpha hydroxy acid on your skin, using a moisturizer, not smoking and having abnormal skin growths removed. Even though you do all those things, laser skin resurfacing is still a useful weapon in the battle of aging.

Understand the concept of maintaining your appearance for the rest of your life. You'll find it comforting when you perform the necessary steps. Think of laser skin resurfacing as being one of the available steps to take. In the future you'll find people having laser skin resurfacing at even younger ages than those who are doing it now. It makes sense for someone who has a youthful appearance to maintain it and not allow it to be lost by the aging process. Why should movie stars be the only ones to understand this and seek this out?

A women in her mid-thirties who sees fine wrinkles around her eyes won't want to wait until the age of forty-five to first try to improve her appearance. The aging effect on her skin is already apparent. She doesn't want to let this go untreated for ten years when treatment that can help is available now. Men can benefit from this as much as women. In the future you'll find more and more people having repeat treatments with laser skin resurfacing because of the good it does.

Laser skin resurfacing is helpful for more than treating fine wrinkles that occur with aging and blotchiness. It can also treat precancerous conditions of the facial skin. A precancerous condition of the skin means that the person has been identified to have many growths of the facial skin that, left untreated, can lead to skin cancer. I have patients in my practice who have undergone laser skin resurfacing of the entire face for this very reason. The treatment significantly removes the superficial layer of the skin that contains certain precancerous growths. The entire facial skin which has been laser skin resurfaced will now have a more youthful appearance. No matter what the reason is for having laser skin resurfacing, your skin will benefit from it.

75.

Chemical Peels Can Also Be Used To Treat Fine Wrinkles And Blotchiness Of The Facial Skin

Chemical peels of the facial skin involve agents like trichloroacetic acid (TCA), phenol and other products. You cannot purchase these chemicals for your own use at home. Chemical facial skin peels must be done only under the supervision of a doctor. It would be dangerous for you to have this done any other way. Specific concentrations of each chemical must be used to maximize the safety and its effect.

A trichloroacetic acid peel or TCA peel involves applying a specific concentration of trichloroacetic acid on the skin. The acid affects the skin by peeling away the superficial layer. The higher the concentration of the trichloroacetic acid used, the deeper the peel of the skin. The deeper the peel, the more successful the improvement of fine wrinkles. Too superficial of a peel will not result in any significant improvement. Too deep a peel can lead to delayed healing and scarring. A TCA peel will not give as deep a peel as laser skin resurfacing or phenol, but it can remove fine wrinkles, help blotchy skin look more uniform in appearance and lead to a smoother skin. A TCA peel is applied once and then the skin is allowed to peel and heal. Repeat treatments can be done but usually not until months or years have passed.

The phenol peel involves applying phenol (another acid) on the skin. A phenol peel works in the same way as a TCA peel, and varying the concentration of the phenol has the same effect as varying the concentration of the TCA. A phenol peel helps treat fine facial wrinkles, smooths the skin and makes it look less blotchy, just like a TCA peel. However, the phenol may lighten the treated skin more than a TCA peel or laser skin resurfacing. Unlike TCA, the phenol agent can also cause heart irregularities if too much is applied at once. Phenol is not as commonly used today as in the past. It's been replaced in many instances with laser skin resurfacing because laser skin resurfacing technology allows for a more accurate depth of penetration of the skin surface than acids do.

Two to four days after these chemicals are applied, the superficial layer of the skin will blister and start to peel off, continuing for another week or two. A new superficial layer of fresh skin will grow in its place. The skin's appearance at the first week following a chemical peel is similar to the appearance of skin following a laser skin resurfacing. After healing occurs the skin treated with a chemical peel will have a smoother, more glowing color. Blotchy skin and fine wrinkles will also be improved.

Chemical peels can be done under local anesthesia, intravenous sedation, where an I.V. is started and medicine is given to make you sleepy, or under general anesthesia. Complications include but are not limited to infection, bleeding, scarring, and color change. A chemical peel can be repeated in the future although an appropriate amount of time is needed between any retreatment.

Cover makeup can be applied once the skin heals. It may help blend in coloration between treated and untreated skin. It's very important to protect the skin from sunburn after chemical peel or after laser skin resurfacing. Makeup with sunblock is beneficial. As the technology of laser skin resurfacing continues to progress, chemical peels will play a less prominent role. Chemical peels will, however, always have their place in the realm of skin care.

76.

Renova Cream

Renova is a form of vitamin A available only by a doctor's prescription. The direct effect of Renova on the skin is to cause the skin to have a smoother and more youthful appearance. Renova comes as a cream and is applied directly on the facial skin before bedtime. A similar product, Retin-A, is used for acne and to help smooth the skin.

Women who are pregnant or women who can possibly become pregnant must not use Renova because this vitamin A product can harm a developing fetus. A patient must not share Renova with anyone. I have to instruct my female patients who are in their fifties and sixties not to let their daughters use it because they might be pregnant or have the potential to become pregnant.

The patients who try to share their Renova don't understand the dangerous effect it can have on a fetus. The safest thing to do with any prescription medication is to never share it with others. You can't possibly understand all the dangers of a prescription medication, especially if you let others use it.

The most appropriate time for applying Renova is every night at bedtime for the first year. This allows it to work through the night on the facial area. Its potency can be decreased by sunlight so nighttime use is ideal. Anyone using Renova must not sunburn. Sun protection is necessary because Renova will cause your skin to be more sensitive to the sun's harmful effects. If someone develops too much skin sensitivity, however, then they may need to stop using it. It's important to know that the skin sensitivity reaction may go away on its own even if the Renova is continued. A steroid cream can be applied to the skin to help during this time.

The effect of the Renova may not be apparent for four months and it can take as long as one year. If someone develops a skin irritation during the initial use of the Renova, there can be some skin swelling. This temporary skin swelling will make the fine wrinkles less apparent. When the swelling improves the fine wrinkles will reappear. Realize that the improvement of facial wrinkles was due to facial swelling, which is temporary and not a permanent effect of the Renova.

After one year of use the Renova can be tapered to only several nights a week. Renova will not treat significant facial wrinkles but may help the skin appear as healthy as possible. It's important to still continue with the other things that make your facial skin healthy. These include sun protection, not smoking, moisturizing your skin, using alpha hydroxy acids, having facial growths treated and having laser skin resurfacing or chemical peeling when indicated.

77.

Eyelid Puffiness And Bagginess Can Be Improved To Create A More Youthful Appearance

People in their early thirties or younger will start to see signs of aging around their eyes. The upper eyelid skin will develop fine wrinkles and there may be more puffiness in that area than in the past because of fat bulging. People try to pass this off as a result of not getting a good night's sleep but even when they have slept well, the puffiness remains. Excess upper eyelid skin can droop onto and over the upper eyelashes, obstructing vision in some cases. These signs of aging can be improved.

The lower eyelids tend to develop fine wrinkles that later can lead to much deeper ones. Puffiness/bagginess of the lower eyelids due to fat bulging can also occur. The lower eyelid can stretch and weaken, sometimes pulling down and away from the eyes. The lower eyelids can even assume a sunken appearance that wasn't apparent before.

Signs of aging of the upper and lower eyelids are easy to see. They make a person look much older than they actually are. People in their forties with puffy and baggy eyelids may appear to be in their late fifties or sixties. People in their sixties with eyelid bagginess will look even older. The appearance of the eyelids can be significantly improved.

An eyelid lift, also know as blepharoplasty, is performed and the excess skin, muscle and fat are removed. For the upper eyelids the skin incision is placed into the natural upper eyelid skin fold, making the incisions as well concealed as possible. In addition, forehead skin sagging can cause the eyebrows to droop onto the upper eyelids, aging their appearance. To improve this condition, the eyebrows are lifted into a more youthful position. This is called a forehead lift and it can be done at the same time the upper eyelid procedure is done.

For the lower eyelids the skin incision is made immediately below each lower eyelash margin. Skin, muscle and fat excess are removed through this incision. If the lower eyelid needs to be tightened, that can be done at the same time. To avoid a lower eyelid skin incision, an incision can be made on the inside of the lower eyelid. This is called a transconjunctival blepharoplasty. Fat excess can be removed through this incision. At the same time a transconjunctival blepharoplasty is done, the lower eyelid skin surface can undergo laser skin resurfacing to improve the fine wrinkles.

Stitches are placed to close the skin incision and are removed within three to five days. Swelling of the eyelids at this time is normal and usually maximizes by one to three days. Bruising can also be seen around the area but is short lasting. Soon after the stitches are removed, a cover makeup can soon be applied to conceal any bruising. The upper eyelids will appear to be more youthful. They'll have a more open look because the bulging skin, fat and muscle excesses will have been removed. Previous bagginess of the lower eyelids will be lessened by the procedure. When you look in the mirror your attention will not be drawn to your puffy eyelids anymore because they will be improved. The eyelid lift is a very rewarding and common procedure for both men and women. As with any procedure, complications to watch for include but are not limited to infection, bleeding and scarring. The procedure can be done under local anesthesia, intravenous sedation, where an I.V. is started and medicine is given to make you sleepy, or under general anesthesia. Since the incisions are placed in such naturally concealed areas, it may be hard to find them later on. When you look at someone who has had the procedure, you'll only know they look better, more youthful and rested. Botox and injectable fillers can be effective as a non-surgical option. These can also be combined with the surgical option.

78.

Facial Skin Sagging Can Be Improved With A Face-Lift

Gravity has a huge influence on your face, causing the skin to sag down. During your youth your skin had excellent tone and was able to combat the effect of gravity. As the elasticity and tone of your skin decreases with age, the skin cannot successfully fight the pull of gravity and your facial skin moves downward. How well you've protected your skin over the years and your hereditary predisposition to aging also have a bearing on facial skin sagging. With aging the muscles under the facial skin will sag with the skin. Sagging in the cheek region can cause the face to have a more drawn out appearance. By pulling upward and back on the facial skin, you can recreate a more youthful positioning of your skin. Sagging of the facial skin may also be associated with extra fat deposits that were not previously present. Facial skin sagging may exist along with fine or deep wrinkles of the facial skin.

Skin sags downward because people walk upright. If someone walked upside down on their hands all their life, their neck skin would start to sag up over their jaw line and on to their cheeks. This would be the exact opposite of what happens now. If you lived on the moon where the gravitation effect is only one sixth that of Earth, it would have a lesser effect on your skin. The fountain of youth may be found where there is less gravitation effect. If you orbited around the Earth, you'd be in zero gravity and would experience no facial sagging. The only problem with long term zero gravity is that you would lose muscle mass even if you exercised constantly. When you lose muscle mass it's difficult to come back to Earth and walk without a problem. You'd feel like you were carrying around a heavy load. If you could ever spend years on a planet with a much greater gravitation force like Jupiter the aging effect on your skin due to gravity would be even worse than on Earth. Talk to your travel agent. The rule of thumb on interplanetary travel is the greater the gravitational effect, the worse the ultimate skin sagging.

Skin sagging that occurs over the years can be reversed. The skin can be pulled up and back into a more youthful position. The muscle layer below can be tightened in a similar fashion. This is considered a face-lift. Excess fat that existed under the skin could also be reduced at the same time. The face-lift procedure involves an incision from in front of each ear and continuing behind that ear. The incisions are located in a naturally appearing crease in front of the ear, making them as inconspicuous as possible. Depending on how much skin excess needs to be removed, the incisions may be shorter or longer than this. If an endoscope and endoscopic technique is used, the incisions may be even shorter. An endoscope is a lighted scope with a television camera attached to it. The incisions can be closed with stitches under the skin that would not be visible to the eye. In addition, think of your hair as camouflage. The longer a person's hair, the easier it is to conceal the incision sites.

The face-lift procedure is available for both men and women. Following a face-lift the face appears more youthful. Skin tightening also gives a more sharply defined jaw line, reversing the hands of time. With skin sagging improved, you'll feel that you look years younger.

It's critical to not be smoking when you undergo this procedure. Smoking can decrease the healthy blood flow needed for maximum healing. People are able to be up and about very quickly after a face-lift. My patients start showering their hair the very next day. Within a week, with makeup applied, it may be difficult to tell when someone had the face-lift done. Gravity will continue to work on your skin after the face-lift. Stay positive! If the skin needs to be retightened in the future, it can be done but it may be years before this is necessary. As with any procedure, complications to watch for include but are not limited to infection, bleeding, problems with healing and changes in skin sensation or muscle function. The procedure can be done under local anesthesia, intravenous sedation, where an I.V. is started and medicine is given to make you sleepy, or under general anesthesia.

The earlier the skin is repositioned into its more youthful position, the longer you'll be able to see the positive effects from a face-lift. One strategy is to work to maintain your already youthful appearance. With this approach having a face-lift done at an earlier age makes sense. Botox and injectable fillers can be effective as a non-surgical option. These can also be combined with the surgical option. Doing what is necessary to keep your face in the best shape possible will have a significant, positive impact later.

79.

Neck Sagging And Fat Excess Can Be Improved Through A Combination Of Skin Tightening, Muscle Tightening And Liposuction

Sagging of the neck skin can be seen in people in their late thirties. A band of skin, running in an up and down direction, pulls away from the midline of the neck in the Adam's apple region. The band of skin may also contain a band of muscle underneath it. This visible band can continue to worsen and more bands of skin may develop next to it.

A sagging neck appears aged. The previous youthful tight skin starts to lose its tone and the effect of gravity takes its toll on the area.

Skin bands can occur with fat excess of the neck. Fat excess causes an obvious bulge of the neck, much like a turkey gobbler. People who aren't overweight can still have a sizable fat accumulation in their necks. The condition may be hereditary. If you notice a son who has the same fatty appearance of the neck as his mother, he's probably predisposed to having fat accumulate in this area.

People who have fat excess in the neck may look heavier than they actually are. Dieting does not help the appearance of a fatty neck in someone who is already at a good body weight. The fat cells in this case are genetically programmed to keep the fat as long as possible. Even if these fat cells receive a message from the body that fat is needed in the system, these are the last cells to want to release the fat.

Those who've been heavy since childhood and have a fatty neck, however, may be able to improve it with weight loss while they're still young, although the neck will still retain some fat. In virtually all cases a fatty neck appearance does not go away on its own. Fat from the neck must be removed by cutting it out or by using liposuction.

Sagging neck skin and sagging neck muscle can be tightened during a face-lift. It is a normal part of the procedure. The face-lift not only improves the facial skin sagging but the neck sagging as well. The inconspicuous incision around the ear is still the same but a small incision under the neck may be added to complete the muscle tightening. Tightening of the neck skin can create a more youthful look. Lessening the banding of the neck skin can have a dramatic effect on improving your appearance.

Fat excess of the neck can be removed at the same time the face-lift procedure is done. Once the excess fat is gone, the skin will no longer bulge out. Removing fat excess of the neck can have impressive results on one's appearance. Fat excess can be cut away directly or removed by liposuction. These procedures can be done at the same time as the skin tightening. In younger individuals with good skin tone, a fatty neck can be treated with just liposuction and no skin tightening. The skin will contract down over the treated area. When liposuction of the neck is the only procedure performed, a small incision is made behind each earlobe and another one is possibly placed under the chin. An entire neck liposuction can be done in this way.

As with any surgical procedure, complications to watch for include but are not limited to infection, bleeding, scarring and problems with skin healing. The procedure can be done under local anesthesia, intravenous sedation, where an I.V. is started and medicine is given to make the patient sleepy, or under general anesthesia. The effects of aging on the neck can be improved and the fatty appearance of the neck can be corrected. The earlier an aged and fatty neck is treated, the better. The overall result is maximized if treatment occurs when the aging effects are first seen. Botox treatment to the neck muscles (Platysma muscles) may have some benefit as a non-surgical option. These can also be combined with the surgical option.

80.

The Effects Of Aging On The Forehead Skin Can Be Improved

Forehead skin is affected by gravity like the face and neck skin. Over time the forehead skin sags downward and pushes the eyebrows down from their higher, more youthful position. The eyebrows can start to crowd out the upper eyelids, making them look more aged.

Forehead skin also migrates down along the outer corners of the eyes, leading to more prominent wrinkling in this area and eventually to obvious crow's feet. A more aged appearance will result. Not only can the skin sag but deep and fine wrinkles of the forehead skin can occur. The skin may also have a rough texture.

A number of things can improve aging forehead skin. These techniques can be used alone or in combination with each other. To improve wrinkles or a roughened appearing forehead, laser skin resurfacing is a great option. It removes the upper, damaged skin layer of the forehead and gives the area a smoother, softer, less wrinkled, and healthier appearance.

Chemical peel can also be done, using phenol or trichloroacetic acid, but laser skin resurfacing provides a more accurate depth of treatment and may also give a tighter appearance to the skin. If the eyebrows are significantly sagged, however, laser skin resurfacing will not tighten the skin enough to adjust the eyebrows to a more youthful position.

To tighten the forehead skin a forehead lift can be done. In the classic forehead skin tightening, an incision is made in the scalp toward the hairline. It extends from the region of one ear to the other ear. The forehead skin is lifted and pulled upward, excess skin is trimmed off and the incision closed. Skin sagging at the outer corners of the eyes as well as the eyebrows can be improved.

The forehead lift can be done using an endoscopic technique. An endoscope is a lighted tube which is placed through the incision in the hair bearing portion of the scalp. Through this scope a lighted and magnified view of what is at the end of the tube tip can be seen on a television camera. The operation can be done though the endoscope with much smaller incisions than with the classic technique because not as large an incision is needed to see the area being operated on. With a forehead lift, the muscles between the eyebrows that lead to frowning can be removed. This technique accomplishes a number of wonderful things.

If the eyebrows are drooping excessively, instead of trying to lift them by pulling up on the skin from the hairline area, an incision may be made directly above each eyebrow. The excess skin immediately above each eyebrow is then removed, lifting the eyebrows to a more youthful level.

As with any type of procedure, complications to watch for include but are not limited to infection, bleeding, problems with healing and changes in skin sensation or muscle function. The procedure can be done under local anesthesia, intravenous sedation, where an I.V. is started and medicine is given to make the patient sleepy, or under general anesthesia. A forehead lift and laser skin resurfacing can be done at the same time. The benefit of lifting sagging forehead skin via the forehead lift procedure can be combined with the benefit of smoothing the skin surface via laser skin resurfacing. Botox and injectable fillers can be effective as a non-surgical option. These can also be combined with the surgical option.

81.

Wrinkling Of The Skin Between The Eyes Can Be Improved With Botox, Muscle Removal Or Laser Skin Resurfacing

Wrinkles become more evident with aging, especially wrinkles between the eyes and eyebrows. These skin wrinkles are seen where the nose meets the forehead and are oriented vertically or horizontally. They may become more prominent due to the muscle under the skin contracting over the years. There are helpful measures available to improve this. Botox is one such treatment. Removal of the muscle that's responsible for contracting the skin is another treatment and laser skin resurfacing is another option.

Botox refers to botulism toxin and is available by physician use only. Botox can help minimize wrinkles in this area because it stops or decreases muscle contractions. When the muscle doesn't contract, the wrinkle becomes less noticeable. The muscles responsible for a specific wrinkle are injected with Botox. A muscle doesn't stop contracting immediately upon injection, it may take two weeks or more to see any effect, which will then last for up to three months. In order to have the muscle continue to be weakened, it will need to be retreated with Botox every three months.

The Botox comes in a frozen sterile vial. Prior to injection the vial is removed from the freezer, allowing the Botox to thaw out. The vial top is popped opened and sterile saline is added. It's mixed together and the botulism toxin is drawn up into a syringe. A fine needle is placed on the syringe. The area to be injected is prepped with alcohol or betadine and the region to be injected is marked out. The needle is inserted through the skin to the muscle level and the wrinkle causing muscle is injected with Botox. The goal is to inject the entire muscle region so a number of injections are done. There is a limit on how much you can have treated in one session. The forehead area, the crow's feet area (skin at the outer aspect of the eyes), lower eyelids, nose, lips, chin and neck can also be treated with Botox. No anesthesia is needed when the Botox is given.

Although not a common occurrence, sometimes when Botox is injected close to the upper eyelids, it may temporarily cause them to droop. Botox treatment is usually not permanent so it is repeatedly every three months. For a more permanent treatment the muscle that is causing a specific wrinkle can be removed during an upper eyelid blepharoplasty or a forehead lift procedure.

Botox is not only used to decrease muscle contraction. It is also used to decrease perspiration under the arms and on significantly sweaty palms. To produce this result, Botox is injected into the skin in the vicinity of the sweat producing glands. These conditions also require retreatment after three months or longer.

Laser skin resurfacing is another option for treating wrinkles. The treatment works on the superficial skin surface level to soften the wrinkled appearance. Laser skin resurfacing doesn't stop the cause of the wrinkle if it's due to muscle contraction, which is why removal of the muscle is appropriate in selected situations. The direct removal of the muscle can be done at the same time laser skin resurfacing is done or at a separate time. Laser skin resurfacing can be accomplished under local anesthesia, intravenous sedation, where an IV. is started and medicine is given to make the patient sleepy, or under general anesthesia.

Thin Lips Can Be Made Fuller, Thick Lips Can Be Made Thinner

With aging, people who have had normal appearing, full lips may notice that their lips become less prominent. It is normal for the lip fullness to decrease over the years. This may be more noticeable in the upper lip. Other people may have had thin lips since their high school years because they were genetically predisposed to have them from an early age. Both of a person's lips may be thin or only the upper or lower lip. Those who have always had thin lips will still see the effects of the aging process as their lips can continue to get even more thinned out as the years go by. Help, however, is available.

There are a number of procedures to make thin lips appear thicker and fuller. One technique is to inject collagen in the lip region to give it a plumper look. Collagen is very short lasting and may stay for only three months before needing to be repeated. The common collagen used for an injection is derived from purified cow collagen. It's been treated so that there is only a slight chance of an individual reacting to it. A test dose of collagen is first injected into a person's skin in an area hidden from site, usually on the arm. If there is no significant skin reaction after a month, the collagen can be injected into the lip region. You can have your own collagen used by having a segment of your skin removed and sent to a lab. The lab will extract collagen from the skin and ship it back in a syringe. Your own collagen can then be injected into the lip area.

Fat injection is another option. Fat is taken from one area of your body and then injected into the lip region. This is longer lasting than collagen and can last as long as six months. If you have liposuction done to improve your shape, fat will be immediately available to inject into the lips. The fat injection will need to be repeated in the future.

Implants made of artificial material can be placed in the upper lip. A common type of lip implant has the appearance of a long, flexible tube with a small diameter. A small incision is made on the ends of the lip and the implant is then placed along the undersurface of the upper lip, providing fullness.

A more permanent procedure which does not require implants is available. The technique involves rolling out the rest of the lip that is already present but hidden away. The result will be a fuller, more youthful appearing lip. The upper or lower lip or both lips can be treated. The procedure involves making an incision on the inner aspect of the lip in the shape of the letter "W". The incision goes along the length of the lip and will be out of view when you look at the lip. After the incision is made, the lip tissue is advanced and dissolvable stitches are used to close the incision.

The lip is made fuller by rolling and advancing more lip tissue where it is needed. The concept for this is derived from the decades of knowledge gained by plastic surgeons while treating lip deformities resulting from cleft lip and trauma. The significant benefit of this technique is that the result is permanent and doesn't have to be repeated every three to six months like the injection procedures. There is no need for implant material in the lip. This technique can also be reversed. If someone, for whatever reason, no longer wants to have the fuller, thicker lips, the lips can be returned to their previous state. The reality is that after having thin lips, people enjoy having the fullness back to their lips.

An individual who has had too thick of a lip to begin with can have the shape improved. An incision is made on the inner aspect of the lip and excess lip tissue is removed. The lip is rolled in and under to make it less prominent and then the incision is closed with dissolvable stitches. This results in a more refined and thinner appearance of the lip. This can be done for the upper lip only, the lower lip only or both lips at the same time.

With virtually all of the procedures mentioned complications to watch for include but are not limited to infection, bleeding, problems with healing, and changes in skin sensation or muscle function. These procedures can be done under local anesthesia, intravenous sedation, where an I.V. is started and medicine is given to make the patient sleepy, or under general anesthesia. Other injectable fillers are available to make the lips fuller and can be effective as a non-surgical option.

83.

Noses Can Be Reshaped, Nasal Breathing Improved

Noses come in all shapes and sizes. Some people are born with the perfect nose, well proportioned and fitting the rest of their face. Others may have noses with sizes and shapes that are less than ideal. The appearance of their nose may not complement the rest of their facial features. The nose's shape may draw attention to itself or a person may even have difficulty breathing out of their nostrils. In these situations it may be possible to change the shape of a nose so it will be more appealing. This is referred to as a rhinoplasty. Nasal breathing can be helped at the same time the nose shape is improved.

Some people have inherited nose shapes that make them unhappy. They may notice that they have the same type of nose as someone else in their family. An undesirable nose shape can also be the result of an injury, such as a blow to the nasal area. Although not all nose fractures are associated with a change in the nose's original shape, a broken nose can deviate from its normal position. This may be apparent immediately after the injury or the nose may look fine initially and then take on a different, deviated, shape over a period of months. The new deformed shape will not be desirable.

It may be difficult for a person to breath through his or her nose due to a deviated nasal septum. The nasal septum is the partition that separates the left nasal passage from the right nasal passage. The rigid part of the septum is composed of cartilage and bone and is covered by a red lining called the mucosa. A deviated nasal septum can occur when someone is struck in the nose. The septum can fracture or become displaced so that it becomes deviated from the injury. A person can also be born with a deviated nasal septum. A septum can be deviated into both nasal passages or only into the left or right side. It can partially or totally obstruct air flow through each nasal passage. Symptoms will include difficulty breathing out of the involved nostril.

Other problems leading to breathing difficulty can exist within the nasal passage. Small bony structures, called inferior turbinates, grow off the side walls of the nasal passage and are covered with the red nasal lining called mucosa. These bony structures can swell and enlarge, blocking the airflow. Sometimes a person can have airflow problems due to an enlarged inferior turbinate in combination with a deviated nasal septum.

It's common for a teenager to undergo nose reshaping or rhinoplasty. Many older individuals also have their nose reshaping done because their parents didn't make the procedure available to them when they were younger. To reshape a nose, the bone and cartilage under the skin is altered. In general, the upper third of the nose is composed of bone; and the middle third and the lower third, or nasal tip, of cartilage. Bone is hard and immovable but cartilage is pliable and can be bend with finger pressure. In a rhinoplasty, excess bone and cartilage is removed and the remaining bone and cartilage is reshaped to give the nose its final improved appearance. In certain circumstances cartilage or bone may be added to regions of the nose. One example is a type of nose called a boxer's nose that appears to be smashed into the face. Bone or cartilage is added to this nose to build it back up to its original position.

Nostril shape can be improved. If their is wide flaring on the outside aspect of the nostrils this can be improved. A small wedge of skin is removed from each side of the face where the side of the nostril meets the cheek, giving the previously widened nostrils a narrower appearance.

A deviated septum can be improved at the same time as the nasal reshaping. Depending upon its location, the deviated portion of the septum may be due to cartilage only, bone only, or a combination of cartilage and bone. An enlarged inferior turbinate can be reduced in size at the same time.

The objective of the nose procedure is to improve the shape of the nose and improve any breathing problem that may exist. As with any procedure complications to watch for include but are not limited to infection, bleeding, changes in skin sensation and problems with healing. The procedure can be done under local anesthesia, intravenous sedation, where an I.V. is started and medicine is given to make you sleepy, or under general anesthesia. The procedure involves making well concealed incisions on the inside of the nose with a possible small incision on the skin between the nostrils. A cast is placed on the nose at the end of the procedure. A packing may be placed into each nostril but is usually removed at one to three days. Skin stitches are removed within five days and the cast by one week. Within 3 to 4 weeks any swelling and bruising of the nose area may be unnoticeable. In certain cases, injectable fillers may be effective as a non-surgical option.

84.

Ears That Are Too Prominent Can Be Reshaped

Any abnormal shape to the ear will be seen at birth. An infant's ears that are too prominent and stick out too far from the side of the head, will persist a lifetime. Adults who have prominent ears can look at their baby and childhood pictures and notice their ears look the same now as they did then. Abnormally shaped ears will stay unchanged unless something is physically done to try to improve them. The procedure to correct prominent ears is called an otoplasty.

Along with being too prominent, ears can also have unnatural bumps. The shape can be distorted along any or all of the ear, making it appear too large or too small. The unnatural appearance of the ear may be different on one side compared to the other. One ear may stick out from the side of the head more than the other ear and its shape and height may be different. Abnormal skin bulges may also be seen in front of the ear region. Some children are born with virtually no ear but fortunately this is not very common. It is more common to see ear deformities presenting as prominent ears or distorted ears. These more common deformities are usually not associated with any hearing loss.

Children with prominent ears may be teased about their appearance by other children. Many times children will first bring up the issue of their ears with their parents because they're being teased. Parents may try not to say anything about it until they are finally forced to discuss the problem. Using long hair to conceal the shape of the ear is the first step that can be taken. It will help decrease the episodes of other children making fun of them.

There is help for these abnormally shaped ears. The prominent ear can be made less prominent so that it appears normal. The timing of the procedure is important. To correct a prominent ear, it's best to wait until the child is five or six years old. This age is important because by then the ear has already reached 80% of its adult size. It's hard to imagine this but it's true. Waiting until the age of five or six years old can make this operative correction the only procedure necessary for the rest of the child's life. Other procedures of the ears can be done at an earlier age. If there are abnormal skin bumps in front of the ear, these can be removed prior to age five or six. These skin bumps may also contain cartilage which, if present, should be removed along with the skin excess.

Adults who have not yet had their prominent ears corrected can have it done at any time. It's a common procedure for people in their twenties. They realize that they want the benefit of a reshaped ear and don't want to wait any longer. Virtually all the adults wish they had the correction done while they were younger. It may not have been done when they were children because their parents may not have thought it was important to correct. It is also possible that their parents may have wanted them to make their own decision as an adult or there were financial obstacles to consider.

Correcting a prominent ear requires an incision behind the ear. The incision ends up in the groove between the back of the ear and the side of the head. It can be the only incision needed and it is in a very inconspicuous location. After the incision is made on the back of the ear, the cartilage is reshaped by placing permanent stitches through the back of the ear cartilage and under the skin. When these stitches are tied down they reshape the ear cartilage. Excess cartilage on the back of the ear might also be shaved down. The ears will be closer to the side of the head and have a more normal appearance. The excess skin on the back of the ear is removed and the incision is closed with dissolvable stitches under the skin. No visible stitches will be seen and no skin stitches will need to be removed.

Other deformities of the ear may be able to be treated at the same time. A bulging and prominent earlobe can be corrected with an incision behind the earlobe that will make it less prominent and more natural appearing. As with any procedure, complications to watch for include but are not limited to infection, bleeding and problems with healing. The procedure can be done under local anesthesia, intravenous sedation, where an I.V. is started and medicine is given to make you sleepy, or under general anesthesia. Following the reshaping procedure a dressing is applied to the head to cover the ears. It is removed within three to five days. It's important to wear a head band at bedtime for up to three weeks to cover and protect the ears.

85.

Chins Can Be Made More Prominent

On side profile a normal projecting chin will have a more pleasing appearance than a receding chin. A receding chin is caused by a lack of adequate outward projection from the jaw bone at the chin level. Help is available. A receding chin can be associated with the upper and lower teeth not fitting together properly; a condition called malocclusion. On profile, a pleasing chin projection will usually be seen to line up within the straight lines which are dropped from the front end of the lower lip and the front end of the upper lip. You need to use two mirrors to be able to see your side profile in this way. Receding chins can be made more prominent through a procedure is called a chin augmentation.

An implant can be used to create the necessary projection. The implant can be made out of a number of different materials and can come prefabricated, already having the desired shape and projection. Other implants need to be shaped and molded at the time they are placed in. After an incision is made under the chin or on the inside of the mouth, the implant is placed into position against the chin bone. Artificial implants work very well for most corrections.

If a significant amount of projection is needed then a different procedure may need to be done. For a greater amount of chin projection, a cut is made on the chin bone and the lower portion of the bone is slide forward, like a drawer to increase projection. The advanced bone is held in place with permanent wires or screws and plates. These wires, screws or plates are under the skin and out of sight.

A person may have a receding chin and malocclusion. In certain circumstances an operation is needed to correct both conditions. The jaw bone and the bone containing the upper teeth (the maxilla) may need to be moved in relation to one another to get the teeth to fit together again. The receding chin can be improved at the same time that the malocclusion is treated but this involves a more complex procedure. The operation would allow normal chewing to occur again and also give a more pleasing chin projection.

A nice chin profile gives a more pleasing look to the overall facial appearance. With any procedure, complications include but not limited to infection, bleeding, changes in skin sensation and problems with healing. A chin augmentation can be done under local anesthesia, intravenous sedation, where an I.V. is started and medicine is given to make a patient sleepy or under general anesthesia. A receding chin will often be treated in combination with a nose reshaping procedure. The overall improvement can be outstanding! With the placement of a chin implant, recover is quick and the results are immediate.

86.

For Women, Breasts That Are Too Large Can Be Made Smaller And The Symptoms Related To Large Breasts Improved

A woman can develop large breasts at different decades of her life. Some women get significant enlargement of their breasts while still in grade school and high school. By the time they are out of high school, they have enormous breasts. Others may see their breasts enlarge at a later age. A weight gain over the years may cause the breasts to become larger. Breasts that are too large can cause many symptoms. They make it difficult for a woman to jog or run, partly because of the discomfort felt in the breast area during these activities.

Help is available. Breasts can be made smaller and more in proportion with the rest of the body by a procedure called a breast reduction. Large drooping breasts can be reduced and lifted back into a more youthful position. Women who have large but different sized breasts can have them reduced so they are both more similar in size. Women will find that symptoms of discomfort caused by large breasts are lessened and that it's much easier to fit into clothing.

Many different symptoms can be caused by large breasts. A woman may experience only one, some or all of these. Starting at the top of the body and working down, the first symptom is headache. People may not even realize it but there is a specific type of headache related to large breasts called a frontal headache. A frontal headache causes painful discomfort across the forehead area. This is different from a migraine headache where the symptom is head pain and flashing lights. A frontal headache is muscular in origin and involves the main forehead muscle, known as the frontalis muscle. The frontalis runs in an up and down fashion on your forehead and is responsible for making your eyebrows raise. Large breasts pull on the chest skin, which transmits pull and tension up along the neck, onto the face and finally onto the forehead muscle. I have many patients who have found relieve from these types of headaches after breast reduction.

One patient's neurologist (a doctor specializing in the nervous system) had given her medication to treat her frontal headaches for over three years. I performed a breast reduction on her and after she recovered, she noted that her frontal headaches were gone. She was able stop her headache medication completely. There are obviously other reasons for frontal headache but in specific situations where a patient has large breasts as well as frontal headaches, help may be available through breast reduction.

Women with large breasts may experience neck pain. Shoulder strap grooving and discomfort can occur because the excessive weight of large breasts exerts a lot of pull downward on the bra straps. The chest and breast area can suffer pain caused by the weight of the breasts pulling and stretching down from the chest.

Bras available for large breasts have an underwire support in them that can dig into the undersurface of the breast area and causes pain. A skin rash can occur under the breasts. Back pain is common, and may be confined to the upper back, mid back or lower back or may run along the entire length of the back. In some cases numbness of the little finger occurs when large breasts cause a pull on the nerve in the armpit area that provides sensation to the little finger. Breasts that are very large tend to sag significantly. It is common to see breasts that sag all the way to a women's belly button.

Breast reduction is the answer to these problems. A woman can go home the same day of the procedure or stay overnight in the hospital. Incisions can vary but are typical located along the crease under the breast (called the inframammary fold), around the pigmented region of the areola and from the bottom of the areola to the breast crease. The nipple and areola are usually left attached to the gland tissue of the breast to help maximize the sensation of the nipple and areola later. Women who have a breast reduction done before they have children may still have the ability to breast feed because the nipples still have connections to the breast gland.

Breast reductions can be offered to women starting in their teens. Women in their sixties can have a breast reduction. One of the most common statements a patient makes to me after their breast reduction is that she should have had the treatment years earlier. A woman in her forties who has had symptomatic large breasts since her high school years has suffered for over twenty years. After the breast reduction she will realize that she did not have to suffer from the symptoms for all those years.

Complications to watch for include but are not limited to infection, bleeding, problems with healing and changes in skin sensation. The procedure can be done under intravenous sedation where an I.V. is started and medicine is given to make the patient sleepy or under general anesthesia. It is common for a woman to resume strenuous activity within three to four weeks after a breast reduction. By that time the previous symptoms related to large breasts may not be noticed. The breasts will be smaller and lifted. It will be easier to shop for clothing once the breasts are in better proportion with the rest of the body.

87.

For Women, Small Breasts Can Be Enlarged, Sagging Breasts Lifted

Whether a woman's breasts are too small is her own personal opinion. A women who wears an A cup sized bra may feel her breasts are too small while another women who wears a C cup sized bra can may also feel her breasts are too small even though she wears a C cup bra. On the other hand, a different women who wears an A cup bra may feel her breast size is just right. For those who feel their breast size is just right, enlarging the breasts is not an issue. For those who would like to enlarge their breasts, regardless of their current bra size, help is available. Breasts can be made larger with a breast enlargement procedure.

Breast sagging is another issue. Sagging of the breasts can occur whether women feel their breasts are too small or just right. A women may be happy with her current breast size but not like the way her breasts sag. Obviously, very large breasted women commonly experience sagging because the weight of their breasts pulls the breasts down.

Many different possibilities exist for women requesting breast enlargement. One scenario is a woman who has small breasts that have remained the same size since her high school years. Another scenario is a woman who started with larger breasts but noticed a decrease in her breast size following her pregnancies. Her resulting breast size is smaller and more saggy than she's used to. Another scenario is a woman who has uneven small breasts with one breast an entire cup size different than the other breast.

A breast enlargement procedure is known as a breast augmentation or breast enhancement. A breast enlargement involves making a pocket under the breast tissue and placing a breast implant into that space. The end result is a larger breast. A breast that is also sagging can be made less saggy by increased its size. No other correction of a sagging breast may be needed in these cases. If excess sagging is still present after the breasts are enlarged, then a breast lift procedure can be done at the same time.

The incision for the breast enlargement procedure can be either under the armpit, around the edge of the areola of the breast, at the bottom of the crease of the breast or at the belly button area. The use of an endoscopic technique can aid in creating the implant pocket. An endoscope is a lighted tube with a camera attached. The endoscope is placed into the pocket. By looking at a television screen, the surgeon can see a magnified view of the pocket and continue with the operation.

An implant placed immediately below the breast tissue is called a subglandular implant. An implant placed one level lower, under the muscle in the area, is called a submuscular implant. When an implant is specifically placed only under the pectoralis major muscle, it's referred to as a subpectoral implant.

The implant is composed of an outer shell or envelope made of silicone. The envelope's inner space can be filled with saline, silicone gel or a combination of the two. Currently, saline filled implants and silicone gel implants are available.

What about mammogram testing before the procedure? A women who has no personal history of breast problems, no family history of breast cancer and who has no abnormal findings on a breast exam will not need a mammogram prior to a breast procedure, unless the women has reached the age of thirty-five to forty. Above that age a routine preoperative mammogram is recommended even with no previous history of breast problems.

For the first several weeks after a breast enlargement the breast area will feel tight. The tissue around the implant will continue to relax and feel more comfortable week by week. It may take up to a month before regular exercising is resumed. Regular self breast exams should continue after this on a monthly basis. Monthly self breast exams should be conducted by all women. That includes those with and without implants. Follow-up mammograms are done based on the person's age and depending on her personal medical history. Complications following the operation include but are not limited to infection, bleeding, changes in skin sensation, deflation of the saline implant, rupture of a silicone implant and the need to loosen the pocket in which the implant sits if the pocket tightens more than expected at a later time. The implants may need to be changed in the future. The procedure can be done under intravenous sedation where an I.V. is started and medicine is given to make you sleepy or under general anesthesia. Women are usually very pleased with the results and are happy to have had the opportunity to enlarge their breast size.

A breast lift procedure is available for someone who doesn't want to increase the size of her breasts but just wants to improve the sagging. The concept of the breast lift is to tighten the skin envelope around the breast. The extent of the incisions will depend on the significance of the drooping. For a small amount of drooping an incision around only the areola may be sufficient. For more severe drooping incisions similar to a breast reduction procedure may be needed. Complications to watch for include but are not limited to infection, bleeding, problems with healing and changes in skin sensation. The procedure can be done under intravenous sedation where an I.V. is started and medicine is given to make you sleepy or under general anesthesia. The healing time and complications to watch for are similar to the breast reduction procedure.

88.

Breast Reconstruction Can Create A New Breast, Replacing What Has Been Lost Due To Cancer

Breast cancer can occur in over ten percent of the population. It's possible to beat breast cancer, with early detection the key to successful treatment. The earlier a breast cancer is identified the better. Once identified, there are different treatment options available. Removal of the entire breast is not always the only option. If removal of the breast is required, breast reconstruction is available.

A routine program for breast care should consist of a breast self breast exam once a month after the menstrual cycle, a yearly physical exam by a physician and routine mammograms. The first mammogram is recommended at age thirty five to forty. It will be done earlier than that if a breast lump is discovered during a physical exam before that age. A mammogram can be repeated every year, every other year, or at some other time interval. How frequently it is repeated depends on the person's age, medical history and physical exam findings.

The type and size of the breast tumor are some of the primary factors that determine what type of treatment will be recommended. If a breast cancer is identified early, one option for treatment is a lumpectomy in which more breast tissue is removed around the biopsy site that was identified as cancer. The entire breast is not removed in this breast sparing type of treatment. A lumpectomy is combined with radiation therapy, which follows the operation. Another treatment option is removal of the entire breast, which may or may not be combined with radiation therapy. Radiation therapy, if needed, is started weeks after the operation. The need for chemotherapy will also be assessed.

If a lumpectomy is done and there is no significant change in shape or size to the breast and the nipple and areola are not involved, breast reconstruction is not necessary. In some situations the nipple/areola area is removed during the lumpectomy. If the breast size has not been changed, then breast reconstruction is available to recreate only the missing nipple and areola. If a mastectomy is done and the entire breast is removed, then breast reconstruction is available to recreate the breast mound and recreate a nipple and areola. In some situations both breasts must be removed and both sides reconstructed.

When the entire breast is removed, different options are available to recreate a new breast. First, a new breast mound must be made. One option is tissue expansion, in which an inflatable balloon or tissue expander is placed under the muscle of the breast region. The balloon is inflated with saline (salt water) once a week for up to six to eight weeks, creating a new breast mound. The tissue expander is then replaced with a permanent implant. Certain tissue expanders can be left in place and are considered permanent implants.

Another option for creating a new breast mound involves moving skin, fat and muscle from the lower abdomen to the breast area. This is called a TRAM flap. In this procedure the skin and fat which would typically be discarded in a tummy tuck procedure is used instead to create a new breast mound. The skin and fat still have a blood supply connected to them via the muscle. The muscle is left attached to the undersurface of the fat and skin. In this technique an implant is not needed. Other options exist for creating a new breast mound. After a new breast mound is created a new nipple and areola can be made at a later time. Several methods of creating a new nipple and areola are available.

As with any procedure complications to watch for include but are not limited to infection, bleeding, problems with healing and deflation of the tissue expander or saline implant. The procedure can be done under intravenous sedation where an I.V. is started and medicine is given to create a sleepy state or under general anesthesia. Breast reconstruction can be started at the time the breast is removed or it can be done in a delayed manner. After the new breast is created, the opposite breast may need to be altered in size and shape to match. The opposite breast may need to be reduced in size or lifted or enlarged if it is noticeably different than the reconstructed breast. Breast reconstruction is available to create a new breast, replacing what has been lost due to cancer.

89.

For Men, Large Breasts Can Be Reduced

Starting toward the end of grade school and into the early years of high school, a boy may experience breast development. The breasts will be larger than what would be expected, this condition is called gynecomastia. It commonly occurs because an adolescent boy's breast glands are highly sensitive to the estrogen hormone that is circulating through their system. The estrogen hormone stimulates the breast gland to enlarge. Help is available for teenagers and adults with large breasts.

A physical exam is required to make sure the male breast enlargement is not being caused by other conditions. For example, a doctor will check for the presence of a tumor of the testicle which, though an uncommon reason, could cause breast enlargement. An overweight boy can also have breast enlargement because of excess fat deposited in the breasts and not just breast gland development. Breast enlargement can occur in adult men even though it was not present during their teenage years. There are other reasons this can occur. Certain doctor prescribed drugs can cause breast enlargement, as can the drug, marijuana. Liver damage from excess drinking can also result in enlarged breasts.

One or both breasts may be affected. Men seeking treatment most commonly have both breasts reduced at the same time. In a majority of cases men who have their large breasts made smaller noted that their breasts had appeared large to them since their early teens. They had been embarrassed by their breasts for all those years. It was especially painful for them to change their clothes in gym class or shower around other boys.

The size of the breasts may get so large that they sag. Help is available for boys and men with enlarged breasts. In males, the feel of the breast tissue can vary. Enlarged breasts may have a relatively soft feel to them, in which case, these soft areas of the breasts are mostly fatty in composition. The breast may also have a very rock hard feel, like feeling a small dinner plate under the breast skin. The firm areas represent the breast gland tissue enlargement. A combination of soft and hard areas may be noticed.

One treatment involves liposuction, which works best on breasts enlarged primarily by excess fat. Several small incisions are made in the breast area and the fat excess is removed. However, for breasts enlarged from breast gland excess, a direct cutting out of the excess breast tissue, called a subcutaneous mastectomy, may be the most effective treatment. The procedure typically involves making an incision at the lower junction of the areola. The breast gland excess is then removed from underneath the skin. If a significant amount of excess breast skin is present, it may need to be removed, requiring a longer incision on the breast skin.

An endoscopic technique can be performed, placing the incision near the armpit and not on the breast skin. A combination of liposuction and direct excision of the breast tissue excess can also be done. The optimal technique can be determined at the time the breasts are examined.

As with any procedure, complications include but are not limited to infection, bleeding, problems with healing, and changes in skin sensation. The procedure can be done under intravenous sedation where an I.V. is started and medicine is given to make you sleepy or under general anesthesia. After the treatment the breast will be flatter and have a more masculine appearance. It may take up to a month before strenuous activities are initiated. The chest area will look more appealing both in and out of clothes.

90.

Sagging Upper Arms Can Be Tightened

The skin of the upper arms loosens as a person ages. Previous firm upper arms will become less firm. If a person moves his or her arms like that of a musical conductor, the skin will swing in one direction while the rest of the arm moves in the opposite direction. There can be excess fat on the arms as well as loose skin. Another presentation is that the upper arms will have significant fat excess but not loose skin. The fat excess may have been present since teenage years; or the arms may have been thin for many decades with the fat accumulation of the upper arms starting much later in life. Help is available for those with skin and fat excess of the upper arms.

Can exercise cure flabby skin and fat excess of the upper arms? If the skin is truly stretched, it won't firm up even if muscle tone is improved. Fat excess in the upper arm area may decrease only if exercising and dieting results in any weight loss. The fact that a muscle is exercised immediately below an area of excess fat doesn't mean that the fat will go away.

Exercising the muscles of the upper arm will help firm up and tone the muscles beneath the flabby skin. For women, if the upper arm muscles are exercised too much, the arms may appear too bulky because of muscle enlargement. Regardless, it's always important to maintain some sort of physical activity.

In situations where only flabby skin is present, it can be tightened. An incision is made along the undersurface of the upper arm, potentially running from the arm pit to the elbow. The length of the incision can vary and may be shorter. The skin excess is removed and the skin is tightened. Activities can be restarted in a short time. Within a month all the normal activities would be expected to resume.

If skin and fat excess are both present then a similar type of procedure is done. The procedure is called a brachioplasty. "Brachio" refers to the arm and "plasty" refers to changing the shape; so the entire term means "changing the shape of the arm." The incision is made along the undersurface of the upper arm, as it would be for the skin removal procedure. Excess fat is removed along with excess skin of the upper arm and the incision is closed. The upper arm will be tighter and have a more slender appearance.

For situations where there is not significant hanging skin excess but mostly a fatty upper arm liposuction can be performed. The fat excess can be removed through several small incisions. The skin tone should be fairly good if liposuction is the only procedure done. The skin may tighten down after the fat excess is removed and the fullness of the upper arms would be decreased. A compression garment is worn over the treated area for up to three to four weeks. A combination of liposuction and removal of skin excess is also possible.

Bruising and swelling are seen but continue to improve week by week. As with any procedure, complications to watch for include but are not limited to infection, bleeding, problems with healing and skin sensation changes. The procedure can be done under intravenous sedation where an I.V. is started and medicine is given to make the patient sleepy or under general anesthesia. The recovery from the liposuction will probably be quicker than from the procedure in which the skin and fat is removed using longer incisions. With time a more attractive appearance of the upper arm will be seen. It's important to maintain a proper diet and workout routine. If this is done, body weight won't increase and the upper arm muscles will stay firm.

91.

Fat Excess Of The Abdomen Can Be Decreased With Liposuction

Your abdomen, or tummy region, extends from your rib cage to your pubic region. The upper abdomen is the area from the rib cage to the belly button and the lower abdomen extends from the belly button down to the pubic region. Immediately below the skin on your abdomen is a fat layer that can be treated during liposuction. Below the fat layer is a muscle layer. The thicker your fat layer, the fatter the area will appear. The fat layer varies in thickness around the abdomen. It's common to see a thicker amount of fat in the lower abdomen. The upper abdomen can also have a thick amount of fat but it may not be as thick as the lower abdomen.

Areas of fat excess on the sides of the lower abdomen have their own nickname. These are the dreaded love handles. One comedian commented that his loves handles were so large that they were called love suitcases. The thickened fat layer on the front and sides of the abdomen can be improved with liposuction.

Are there ways to reduce the thickness of the fat in the abdomen or tummy region other than with liposuction? Weight loss will decrease the overall appearance of excess body fat, but one of the last areas to show improvement with weight loss is the abdomen. There is a genetic predisposition for the fat cells in the abdominal region to hold onto the fat they have collected. Even though these fat cells receive a message from your body to release the fat back into the system, they are unwilling to do so. You may need to get at or below your ideal body weight to finally see the fat excess of the abdomen go away with weight loss. Many people who work out constantly and who are at good body weights still can't reduce the fat excess of their abdomens.

The same thing is true for love handles. Even with diet and exercise, love handles may not change in appearance. With exercise you will be able to firm up the abdominal muscles that are below the fat layer. A firmer and more muscular abdomen will be a bonus. Because you can exercise the abdominal muscles that are immediately below the fat doesn't mean that the thickness of the fat layer will decrease.

You don't need to be at your ideal body weight to have liposuction. A person can weigh over two hundred pounds and still receive significant benefits from liposuction. I have patients who tell me that even though they may consider themselves to be large to begin with, they still appreciate the benefit they have received from liposuction. Yes, they may be large but they feel they look great after the liposuction.

Liposuction is a wonderful option for treating fat excess of the entire abdomen including the upper abdomen, lower abdomen and the love handles. Isolated areas like the love handles or the lower abdomen may be the only areas that need the procedure. Liposuction involves making very small incisions on the abdomen. To make them inconspicuous, the incisions are placed around the belly button and low on the abdomen by the pubic region. If there are previous scars on the abdomen, the incisions can be made at the already present scar sites.

I am always amazed at how much improvement can be made to such a large area through such a tiny incision. A fluid containing medication to decrease blood loss is injected into the fat layer through the incisions. This method is called the tumescent technique of liposuction. It allows for the removal of the greatest amount of fat in the safest possible way. A medication to reduce discomfort can also be added to the injected fluid.

Like any other procedure, complications to watch for include but are not limited to infection, bleeding and problems with healing. The procedure can be done under local anesthesia, intravenous sedation, where an I.V. is started and medicine is given to make you sleepy, or under general anesthesia. A compression garment, like a girdle, is worn over the treated areas following liposuction. It's important to wear this virtually all the time, even at bedtime, for up to three weeks. This helps to decrease swelling to a significant degree. The garment is taken off for daily showering and it can be readjusted throughout the day. Day by day, week by week you will feel better. You want to wait three to four weeks before restarting your full range of strenuous activities. The previous fat bulging will be reduced and the appearance improved.

92.

Excess Skin And Fat Rolls Of The Lower Abdomen Can Be Removed With A Tummy Tuck

Excess skin and fat rolls can be seen on the abdomen, especially the lower abdomen, which is from the belly button down to the pubic area. Skin and fat rolls can also be seen on the upper abdomen, which is located from the rib cage to the belly button. Skin and fat rolls exist for many different reasons. After massive weight loss or after pregnancy, a roll of skin and fat can hang over a person's belt buckle. A skin and fat roll can develop with weight gain. A person may have slender legs and not be heavy, yet they have a significant amount of skin and fat excess of the lower abdomen. When there is significant skin hanging over the belt buckle, exercise will not tighten up the skin. What can be done?

A tummy tuck, also known as an abdominoplasty, can help eliminate the excess skin and fat roll. Liposuction alone doesn't improve this significant skin looseness or excess. The tummy tuck procedure removes the hanging excess skin and fat. It's like a face-lift on the tummy. If needed, the covering over the abdominal muscles can be tightened during a tummy tuck. The appearance of the abdomen will be improved and it will look tighter.

Abdominoplasty means abdomen reshaping. An incision is made along the bikini line on the lower abdomen. It's made as low as possible so it can be concealed by undergarments that are worn later. The skin and fat is then lifted off the muscle covering of the abdomen and then pulled down like a shade. The excess skin and fat is removed. Some individuals who undergo the tummy tuck procedure may primarily have skin excess but not much fat excess, while others have a significant amount of fat being removed at the same time as the skin excess.

The incision along the bikini line is closed. An incision is usually placed around the belly button as part of the procedure. The skin and fat rolls will be eliminated and a tighter abdomen will result. Drains are placed under the skin and removed later, some fluid may collect under the skin after the drains are removed, but it can easily be eliminated. It is important to wait at least a month before resuming any strenuous activities. This will allow enough time to let everything settle down. The skin of the abdomen will feel tight after the procedure. It will continue to soften and feel back to normal week by week. Complications include but are not limited to infection, bleeding and problems with healing. The procedure can be done under local anesthesia, intravenous sedation, where an I.V. is started and medicine is given to make you sleepy, or under general anesthesia.

If fat excess remains after the tummy tuck, it can be liposuctioned at a later time. It's possible to have liposuction done on the abdomen at the same time as a tummy tuck. The extent of the liposuction must be tailored for each individual to determine what can be done safely. Liposuction can be done on the thighs and other areas at the same time as a tummy tuck.

Women are not the only ones who have tummy tucks. Men who are overweight and then undergo massive weight loss can find significant skin and fat excess hanging over their belt buckles. The tummy tuck procedure is the same for both women and men.

People don't have to be at their ideal body weight to have tummy tucks. Many are at least twenty pounds or more over their ideal body weight when they have their tummy tucks. Patients have told me that though they were overweight to begin with, they felt great and thought they looked great because of their tummy tucks. The tummy tuck procedure is a wonderful way to improve the excess skin and fat rolls of the abdomen.

93.

Bulging Thighs Can Be Reduced With Liposuction

A person may have had bulging thighs since high school or their thighs may have become more prominent later in life, possibly associated with weight gain. A person may be at an ideal body weight and work out frequently but still have bulging thighs. Thighs may bulge on the outer aspect of the leg, on the inner aspect or the bulging may wrap around the entire leg. Bulging thighs can be improved. Liposuction can reduce the excess fat that causes the bulging. By reducing the fat excess below the skin level, the skin will come closer to the body. A slimmer and more attractive appearance will result.

People can usually recall when their thighs became too bulging. It becomes apparent when the thigh contour of the leg is first seen to stick out beyond an appealing straight line. Compressive panty hose can help push in the bulging but will not eliminate them.

Certain individuals are predisposed to gaining a lot of their weight in the thigh region. In this situation it's best to maintain a proper weight so the appearance of the thighs is not worsened. If a ten pound weight gain is associated with a significant worsening of the thigh bulging, be aware of this. Know ahead of time that you are doing wonders to maintain your shape by not gaining additional weight.

If those who are overweight can lose weight, there may be an improvement in the general appearance of their thighs. The areas of bulging, however, would not be entirely eliminated. Thigh bulging that is still present after weight loss can be helped with liposuction.

Someone who is at their ideal body weight can have bulging thighs. If someone works out at least three times a week and are at a good body weight, their thigh bulges may not go away. The fat cells in these areas are genetically predisposed to keep the fat in their cells for as long as possible. Even though these fat cells receive a signal from the system to release the fat, they do not do so. Liposuction is the solution in these regions of fat bulging that are unresponsive to a program involving a maintained weight loss through proper diet and exercise.

A very common area to see bulging is on the outer thigh. The outer thigh can bulge along with the upper inner thigh. It is less common to see someone who has bulging of only the upper inner thigh while the outer thigh is not affected. The front and back of the thigh can also bulge from fat excess.

Liposuction is an ideal procedure to help reduce the fat excess in these areas. Only one tiny incision may be needed to treat a specific area, although more than one incision can also be used. The fat excess is then removed with liposuction. More than the outer and upper inner thighs can be liposuctioned at the same time. If indicated, the front and the back of the thigh can be liposuctioned. This is referred to as a circumferential thigh liposuction, which means the liposuction can be done around the entire circumference of the thigh.

Liposuction may also be referred to as liposculpture. Following the liposuction a compressive pair of panty hose or girdle is worn for up to three weeks, even at bedtime. These garments should only be removed when they need readjusting or during showering. It's helpful to have pressure applied to the treated areas to maximize the speed of the recovery and decrease swelling and fluid collection under the skin. It's normal to see bruising in the entire area but this will fade over a period of weeks. As with any procedure, complications to watch for include but are not limited to infection, bleeding and problems with healing. The procedure can be done under local anesthesia, intravenous sedation, where an I.V. is started and medicine is given to make you sleepy, or under general anesthesia.

Within a month strenuous activities can be restarted. Patients will say that they are missing their workout during the recovery time but I tell them not to worry. The improvement they'll see in their appearance from liposuction could not be matched no matter how long they worked out.

94.

A Bulging Buttock And Fat Excess Around The Knees And Calves Can Be Improved With Liposuction

Areas other than the abdomen and thighs can be improved with liposuction. A bulging buttock can be liposuctioned and fat excess around the knees can be treated. It is more common to see fat excess on the inner knees, although there can also be fat excess in front and above the kneecap. Fat excess on the outer aspect of the knee is usually not as pronounced at it is at the inner knee region. The calves can be liposuctioned and fat excess on the back of the calves can be reduced with this method. In addition, other areas, like the upper back where fat rolls may exist, can be treated.

Liposuction to reduce the fat excess at these sites only requires tiny incisions. By pinching the skin before the liposuction, you'll notice a certain thickness between your fingers. This includes the skin and the fat. After liposuction the thickness you pinch will be less because the thickness of the fat layer has been reduced. The end result is that the skin will come closer to the body. It no longer will be plumped out and the bulging appearance it had previously will be reduced.

One female patient who had liposuction of the outer thigh and buttock area was being helped into the shower the next day by her husband. He commented to her how nice it already looked to him from the back. This was only after the first day following the procedure!

Improving the contour of the body through liposuction is a great option. Liposuction is for those areas which can't be reduced by weight loss alone. It's for those areas which don't seem to improve no matter what you've done. When indicated, weight loss can be tried but don't look at weight loss at a temporary fix.

If you're only going to have a temporary weight loss then gain it back this is not helpful. After a failed weight loss people can end up gaining more weight than what they started with. A proper diet and exercise are key components if weight loss is attempted. You need to maintain this as a way of life.

After liposuction of the buttock, knees and calves, a compression garment should be wore for up to three weeks, similar to liposuction of the abdomen and the thighs. The swelling may take a bit longer to improve in the calf area versus the areas above it, simply because it is lower down on the leg. Bruising is normal and may appear purple at first, then change to a green color and finally to a yellow color that eventually fades out. If the bruising initially is a green color, it will fade to yellow and then clear away. The bruising improves over several weeks.

Many regular activities can be started within days, but waiting up to a month before beginning strenuous activities is appropriate. Complications to watch for include but are not limited to infection, bleeding and problems with healing. The procedure can be done under local anesthesia, intravenous sedation, where an I.V. is started and medicine is given to make a patient sleepy, or under general anesthesia.

The goal of the liposuction is to make you look as good as you can. The liposuction can have a very positive effect on your attitude about your body. Patients have told me they feel more confident about their body because of the improvement they see. Not only did it make them look better but it also made them feel better!

95.

Have Any Spider Veins And Varicose Veins Of The Legs Treated

It's very common to see small and large veins come to the surface of the leg skin as a person gets older. Small veins that are usually no wider than the end of a paper clip are called spider veins because they can have a spider like appearance. Varicose veins are much larger and wider and have a rope like appearance. Treatment is available for all of these.

If you think about the appearance of your legs during your teens, you probably won't recall seeing spider veins or varicose veins. Because pregnancy causes an increased pressure on the leg veins, women can develop spider or varicose veins at a much earlier age than their male counterpart.

The increased pressure causes the leg veins and the one way valves within the veins to widen. The one way valves work to allow blood to flow only toward the heart and not back down the leg, but when the valve is widened, it can't close off normally. The blood in the vein will now flow in the wrong direction, back down the leg. This will worsen the condition of the veins even more. This is one cause for varicose veins. Pain and fatigue are associated with varicose veins.

During pregnancy some women will develop both spider veins and varicose veins. This condition may improve after the pregnancy and eventually go away completely, but some women's spider and varicose veins stay and worsen over the years. Wearing compression panty hose is one way to keep the veins compressed down. It helps squeeze the blood out of them, decreasing the pain and fatigue that are experienced when the veins are engorged with blood.

Leg veins are the most engorged when someone is standing. Rest is an important way to relieve this condition, as is elevating the feet as much as possible throughout the day.

Foot elevation allows the blood to drain back to the heart under less pressure. When the varicose veins have less blood pooling in them, there is less pressure. This decreases the pain and fatigue associated with the varicose veins.

Once a varicose vein is present and causing symptoms, treatment should be sought. More than compression and leg elevation are needed. The cause of the varicose vein should be identified by a doctor and the problematic vein corrected.

People are always concerned that eliminating spider veins or varicose veins will cause problems with blood returning to the heart. This is really not true provided a person has a healthy leg and has not had a previous blood clot in the leg. The blood flows primarily up through the leg through veins that are located within the muscles of the legs. Eliminating a superficial leg vein, therefore, would not cause any problems.

The smaller spider veins may or may not be associated with any pain or soreness. These are new abnormal veins and are not part of the original venous system. These new blood vessel growths may not be affected by, or due to, blood back flow. Spider veins can be treated in a number of ways. They can be injected with a medication that will irritate the lining of the vein. This is referred to as sclerosing the vein. The vein will want to close down because of the irritation. The desired result is to have no blood flow through the vein so that it looks as if it disappeared. The vein doesn't close down the moment it is injected. It takes weeks for this to occur.

Laser and radiofrequency devices can also be used for the smaller spider veins. Larger varicose veins require injections of a sclerosing medication along the length of the vein. Multiple treatments, usually once a month, are required regardless of the type of treatment that's done.

Up to four treatments or more at a single location may be needed. If the veins come back, then retreatment is appropriate. For the spider veins compression panty hose should be worn for at least three days; for the larger veins, for up to three weeks. Bruising is normal. It may take months before the ultimate improvement is seen. Some veins need to be physically removed to treat them appropriately. This is commonly referred to as a vein stripping.

When you are having this treatment you should not take any medication that acts like a blood thinner. Aspirin, Motrin, Advil and vitamin E have a blood thinning effect. Coumadin is a pill that is a blood thinner. It's much more powerful than the others just mentioned. These medications will have the exact opposite effect of what you want to accomplish when trying to close off the blood flow through the vein.

Tylenol does not have a blood thinning effect and can be used for pain relief. Stop aspirin, Motrin, Advil and vitamin E two weeks before and two to three weeks after treatment. Complications to watch for include but are not limited to infection, bleeding, and problems with healing. All of the treatments mentioned, excluding the vein stripping, require no anesthesia.

The appearance of the legs and any symptoms of pain and fatigue can improve with treatment. Spider veins and varicose veins that are now present may continue to worsen. To prevent this, have the veins treated. Once you've gotten treatment, work on maintaining your newly improved appearance. It may require more treatments in the future but it will be in your best interest.

96.

Shape The Eyebrow Hairs To Look As Attractive As Possible

Eyebrows are an important feature of your face, so make them as attractive as possible. They may be too thick, or improperly positioned, groomed or shaped. Eyebrow hairs may grow across the middle of the forehead and meet as one continuous strip. If a woman's eyebrows are too thin, she can use a color eyebrow pencil to fill in the area. Don't disregard your eyebrows. An unappealing shape or thickness of the eyebrows should be improved to make you look as attractive as possible. Properly shaped eyebrows can significantly improve your facial appearance.

How close should the eyebrows be allowed to grow together? Look at your face in a mirror. Draw an imaginary line from either the inner corner of the eye or outside edge of the nostril and go straight up to the forehead. This imaginary vertical line is roughly where the eyebrow hair should not cross over. What do you do if the eyebrows cross over this line toward the center of the forehead? Simply use tweezers and pluck out the hairs that cross the line. For men with very thick eyebrow hair at this location, you can use tweezers or an electric shaver. If you use an electric shaver, be careful in this area. You may have to take care of this on a daily basis if you want it to look as neat as possible.

How far out should the eyebrows go? Look again in the mirror. Draw another imaginary line from the outer lower corner of the nose to the outside corner of the eye and beyond. The eyebrow hairs should not go beyond this line as it reaches up on the forehead.

If the eyebrow hairs grow beyond this zone, pluck them with tweezers. It's more common to see eyebrow hairs growing too close together in the middle of the forehead than it is to see them growing too far beyond the outer corner of the eye.

Where should the eyebrows be positioned? The eyebrow arch should not fall below the bony rim of the eye socket. With aging the eyebrow arch can droop below this bony rim and onto the upper eyelids. This lower eyebrow arch would not be considered to be youthful. It's what aging does to your appearance.

An option to correct the eyebrow arch drooping is a forehead lift procedure. It's like a face-lift in that it lifts and tightens the skin but it is done on the forehead skin. The eyebrow arch can be lifted up into a more youthful position. The incision can be placed in the scalp hair to conceal it or at the junction of the top of the forehead and scalp. If the drooping is significant, an incision can be placed closer to the eyebrow skin on the forehead in one of the natural creases there.

Some women will completely shave off their eyebrow hair if it's too low and replace it with an eyebrow pencil liner. For men, this is not a good option. If the lower eyebrow hairs are growing too low and onto the region of the upper eyelids, then use tweezers to pluck out these hairs. This helps make the eyebrows appear less drooping without doing a forehead lift procedure.

What should be the relationship between the inner corner of the eyebrow and the outer corner? Look in the mirror and draw a line from the inner corner of the eyebrow to the outer corner of the eyebrow. They should both be on the same horizontal level. If one edge falls above or below this horizontal line, it can be adjusted. For women, the outer corner of the eyebrow may also be slightly higher than the inner corner of the eyebrow. Pluck out the eyebrow hairs which are going beyond this ideal shape.

Where should the highest point of the eyebrow arch be? Look in the mirror at the colored portion of your eyeball. Find where the outermost region of the colored portion of the eye meets the white of the eye. Draw a line going straight up from this point and onto the eyebrow arch. This is where the high point of the eyebrow arch ideally is located.

Eyebrows should not be too bushy. Pluck the eyebrow hairs to accomplish this. Prevent the eyebrows from showing signs of aging due to color change by plucking out the eyebrow hairs that are graying. The eyebrow hairs can be colored to give them a uniform appearance. For those who have extremely thin eyebrow hairs, you now know how to properly pencil in your eyebrow arch. More youthful, neater and shapelier eyebrows will enhance your overall facial appearance.

97.

Help Is Available For Facial Acne Scars And Chicken Pox Marks

Acne can lead to facial scars either as a single indented facial scar or multiple scars of different depths or sizes. The scars can be distributed equally on both sides of the face or one side can be affected more than the other. Preventing the acne from developing into a severe state is the best way to minimize the risk of scarring, but that's not always possible. Chicken pox can also lead to facial scars. Chicken pox scars are common above the eyebrows and where the forehead meets the nose, but they can occur virtually anywhere in the facial region. The best way to minimize chicken pox scars is to not prematurely remove the scabs that form during a chicken pox outbreak. Even if the chicken pox scabs remain untouched and are allowed to fall off on their own, scarring can still occur. The appearance of the scars from acne and chicken pox may be improved. Treatments include directly excising the pitted scar areas, laser skin resurfacing, dermabrasion, phenol chemical peel and injectable fillers.

Treatments which inject collagen or fat under the pitted scar to plump up the area may not be as successful. The depressed and pitted scar cannot be easily lifted up into the same level as the normal skin. Collagen and fat injections can be tried but are not the first line of treatment and they may be used in conjunction with other more successful treatment options.

Multiple isolated pitted areas of the face can be treated by excising each of these pitted skin regions and then sewing the skin together. A special skin closure can be done so that the stitches that hold the skin together are buried under the skin. No skin stitches would be visible on the surface. The buried stitches would dissolve under the skin and the previous pitted scar would be replaced by normal skin. The crater defect can be improved.

For the first three months following treatment, it's common for the color of the resulting scar to be purple to red and the surface of the incision firm and lumpy. After this time the color usually fades and the firmness softens. It may take several years for this to slowly continue to improve. Cover makeup can be applied while waiting for the color to fade. Sun block is especially important on these treated areas because they are more susceptible to burns from sun exposure than the rest of the skin.

Laser skin resurfacing is another option for treating acne scars and pox marks of the face. The concept is to reduce the surrounding normal skin level to the depth of the pitted or pocked scar. The entire skin region can then heal on a more even level. Laser skin resurfacing can help give a smoother and more uniform appearance to the skin. The laser skin resurfacing is currently the most popular treatment being used. A deep pitted scar may still be seen but will hopefully look less conspicuous. Direct excision of the most pitted scars can be done before the laser skin resurfacing to gain even more improvement.

Dermabrasion works in a similar way to laser skin resurfacing by abrading away the superficial layer of skin. Although a less common treatment option, a phenol chemical peel will also peel away the superficial layer of skin. As with any procedure, complications to watch for include but are not limited to infection, bleeding and problems with healing. These procedures can be done under local anesthesia, intravenous sedation, where an I.V. is started and medicine is given to make the patient sleepy or under general anesthesia. In certain cases injectable fillers may be effective as a non-surgical option. The desired end result is an improved appearance in the facial acne scar or chicken pox mark.

98.

Unwanted Tattoos Can Be Treated

Tattoos are a worldwide phenomenon and have been identified in various cultures for thousands of years. During the Greek and Roman rule thousands of years ago, tattoos were used to mark prisoners. In our culture today people don't have tattoos placed on them unless they want them. The tattoo may tell a story or be a means of expression. It may show patriotism to country or express love for someone.

Some people may have a tattoo that they no longer want. It may no longer express the current feeling they may have for someone or they are simply tired of it. Treatment is available for unwanted tattoos. Cover makeup or laser treatment are options. Directly excising or cutting out the tattoo and closing the skin together is another option but is not as satisfactory as with the laser treatment.

A fast and immediate option for concealing an unwanted tattoo is with the use of cover makeup. The cover makeup color should be as close to the person's natural skin color as possible. The cover makeup is applied directly over the tattoo. This method may not make the tattoo appear invisible but it can help conceal it. The cover makeup should not be a liquid. Liquid cover makeup will streak and not allow for the best concealment. Makeup that is in a paste or powder form is the best option. Paste makeup can come in a lipstick type dispenser or in a small case.

After the makeup is applied directly over the tattoo, it should be blended into the skin with clean fingers. If it comes in a small case, an application sponge may be used to apply it. Some brands of makeup that are designed for the sole purpose of concealing tattoos must be applied in two separate layers.

The first layer may have a green or purple color to it. The second layer is applied over the first and should be a color similar to your skin tone. Read the package information and speak with the people at the cosmetics counter about proper makeup application. The makeup needs to be applied daily to keep the tattoo concealed.

Laser is a wonderful option for improving the appearance of a tattoo. Laser systems are like computers. They are constantly improving. Even though laser systems will be improved in the future, they can be used successfully today. There are laser systems available now that will help. The laser light is directed at the tattoo and the energy from the laser beam travels through the skin surface and strikes the ink pigment. The ink pigment is what makes the tattoo visible on the skin. The ink pigment will microfragment into even smaller particles when struck by the laser light beam.

Once the ink pigment fragments are reduced in size, the white blood cells in the region can eat them. After gobbling up these smaller ink particles, the white blood cells leave the area. If the ink pigment is very superficial in the skin, some of the ink particles may flake off at the skin surface level during healing. The intensity of the ink particles will be reduced. As the ink particles continue to clear, the tattoo will become lighter and lighter.

More than one treatment will be needed to minimize the appearance of a tattoo. It may take at least four treatments to see improvement. This is still an ideal treatment for fading tattoos. One to two months may need to elapse between treatments to allow for the maximum benefit from each treatment.

The final appearance of the tattoo can not always be predicted. Some tattoos will actually seem to have disappeared from site. Others, though they may be significantly lightened, can still be seen when looked for. This is still a great improvement from their originally appearance. Dark colors, including black and red, are some of the most successful colors to be treated with the laser. The ink tattoos that are extremely close to flesh tone skin color are the most difficult.

People who are planning to have a tattoo done by a tattoo artist have asked me what colors are the easiest to treat if they decide in the future that they no longer want their tattoo. A black tattoo would be my answer.

Immediately after the laser treatment the skin may have a white blister look to it. The white blister covers over the tattoo site. The tattoo has not disappeared yet. It is simply under the blister. People are under the impression that the tattoo has immediately disappeared when they look at the skin. I will point out the white blister and explain what has happened. The blister will peel off and the skin will heal within a few weeks.

It takes a month or two to see the benefit from each treatment. Complications to watch for include but are not limited to infection, bleeding, and problems with healing. The procedure can be accomplished using no anesthesia, local anesthesia, intravenous sedation, where an I.V. is started and medicine is given to make you sleepy, or under general anesthesia.

Another method of removing a tattoo is by excising or cutting out the skin that contains the tattoo. The tattoo may be so wide that it's not possible to easily cut out the tattoo and bring the skin back together. Laser treatment is the better option at this time. Even if a tattoo can be cut out and the skin stitched together, the end result may still not be as good as the laser treatment.

What To Do About Nasty Scars

Scars can be the result of many things including an accident, illness or an operation. The appearance of the scar changes over the months and years. Many of the scars fade over time and are less obvious. Scars that heal with uneven edges or look nasty may need to be concealed or retreated. A scar that is discolored can be concealed with cover makeup. Scars should always be protected from sunburn with protective clothing or suntan lotion.

If skin stitches are used to close an opening in the skin, then the stitches need to be removed before they cause visible scarring themselves. You may remember seeing someone's scar and being able to count the stitch marks. Stitches can create a railroad track appearance on the scar itself. The earlier the skin stitches are removed, the better.

In many situations the skin can be closed with dissolvable stitches only under the skin. When I perform face-lifts, breast reductions, tummy tucks and similar procedures, I will use a skin closure technique in which the stitches holding the skin together are hidden under the skin surface.

Plastic surgeons are very adept at this. Eliminating stitch marks across the scar allows for the best appearing scar. Plastic surgeons still use stitches on top of the skin in certain situations, but the concept is to remove them as soon as possible.

What's the natural course of a scar? Initially, it will turn red to purple in color during the first three months, partly due to increased blood flow and to decreased skin pigment. During this time, especially, the scar can also be lumpy and bumpy.

The scar will continue to mature and change over the years. It may take one to two years or more to see the color fade and the scar soften. Some individuals who have thickened scars may have to wait up to five years or more to see their scars soften spontaneously. The softening is a result of the collagen within the scar reorganizing itself. Collagen is the substance that gives strength to the skin.

Many scars fade with time and become very difficult to see. Depending on where the scar is located, it may be easily concealed by clothing. A scar on the scalp, upper forehead or back of the neck can be covered by combing the hair over the area. For elective procedures, plastic surgeons will try to place necessary incisions in inconspicuous locations. If possible, the incisions will be placed along the hair line, within the hair, along skin creases or in directions and locations that will make them difficult to see.

What about those scars that don't fade but tend to look nasty or those that can't be concealed? A scar revision can be accomplished, with three possible results. The revised scar may be better, the same or worse than it was before the revision.

Some scars can be very complex and involved. The scar's size, shape and location all influence how successful a scar revision will be. Scars in different locations on the same person can have different outcomes. A scar on the shoulder may not turn out as well as a scar on the forehead because of the different amounts of tension on the skin in those areas.

A scar that is flat but discolored can be concealed with cover makeup alone. A scar that dips below the normal skin like a crater cannot be concealed as easily with cover makeup, although a very heavy and thick makeup can be used to try to fill in the crater. An injectable filler is an option. This type of scar may need to be revised by removing it and stitching the normal skin edges back together. This procedure may help eliminate the depressed area of the scar. Some scars can be revised with the use of the laser. One option is to laser away the top surface of the scar and the top surface of the surrounding normal skin. After the scar area heals it may blend in better with the rest of the skin.

Pressure can help soften a thickened scar, but it needs to be applied constantly for six months to a year to gain the maximum benefit. A compressive bandage will do the job, especially on the arms or legs. Certain areas of the body like the chest will need a specially fitted garment ordered through a rehab center, physical therapy center or pharmacy.

If the garments are too uncomfortable, the compliance rate for wearing them drops very low over the long term. Compressive garments may be impractical in many circumstances, however, in others they are absolutely necessary.

Injection of a steroid like cortisone into a thickened scar can be tried but is more helpful in treating the symptom of itching of a scar versus its thickening. Radiation therapy to a thickened scar would be a last resort measure.

There are silicone sheets and gels that can be directly applied to the skin to try to soften a thickened scar. To gain the most benefit, these silicone products need to be on the scar virtually all the time, just like the compressive garments. This means they need to be on twenty three hours a day. The one hour they are off during the day is when the patient takes a shower. Silicone sheets and gels must be applied for many months or up to a year to gain the maximum benefit. Options are available for improving the appearance of nasty scars.

100.

Spend Your Youth Attaining Wealth, Spend Your Wealth Attaining Youth

The best time to learn healthy living habits is while you are young. Learn to eat properly and maintain your health. Keep your skin and the rest of your body looking great. It will have a positive impact on you for the rest of your life. Start doing the necessary things which will allow you to feel and look great during your younger years. As you look back on each decade, you'll realize this was the best thing you could have done for yourself.

As you age, you'll see changes that you would like to improve upon. You'll start to see fine wrinkles of the face, fat bulging of the eyelids, fat excess around areas on your body that you may not have seen earlier. Other signs of aging will be present but when you see these changes, you can take action.

You have to budget time into your life to maintain your looks and health. You know that getting your hair styled multiple times each year of your life is part of maintaining your looks. Women who wear cover makeup daily need to factor in that expense. You are already budgeting yourself to maintain your looks? Are you spending the correct amount on yourself or do you need to spend more?

Don't be afraid to spend your wealth to attain youth. Finance it if you want to. It's very similar to remodeling a room in your house. Once the room is remodeled, you're pleased to see the improvement. You still have fond memories of the old room but you're happy with the remodeling. After you see the benefits you receive on attaining youth you will want to maintain this. Think of your face and body as a work in progress.

Attaining and maintaining youth requires a plan. Improve those things that can keep you young. Because of this book you now have a plan laid out in front of you. Use it carefully and wisely. Make the most of your opportunities to feel and look great!

101.

It Is Your Time To Feel And Look Great

Mark the chapters in this book that give you the greatest ideas and suggestions. Turn them into a list of priorities. Put the most important ones at the top of your list. Mark those chapters which give you the most inspiration. Reread all these chapters as many times as possible. Allow these ideas to be the catalyst to making you feel and look great!

Reread this entire book as many times as possible. Depending on where you are in your life, you'll look at certain chapters with new insight as you continue on your road of personal growth and enhancement. You may reread a particular chapter in five, ten or twenty years from now and have a better appreciation of its meaning.

Pay attention to your own needs; otherwise you will not be taking proper care of yourself. Put yourself in a better mood. Be a positive person because it will affect you and others around you in a wonderful way.

With the knowledge of 101 ways to feel and look great, you can organize your thoughts about yourself in a more productive way. It should now be clear to you what you need to do in order to feel and look great. You can go about actually doing it. The knowledge is now in your hands!

*****

101 Ways To Feel And Look Great!

Third Edition

Now is the perfect time for people to reflect upon where they are in their lives, how they feel about themselves, how they look and the state of their health. It is a time for renewed hope and self-improvement.

Everyone in America and the world is focused on the subject of improving one's self. The need to find information on this subject is ever expanding. Also, people are no longer willing to settle for growing old, feeling old or looking old without fighting back. 101 Ways To Feel and Look Great!: A Plastic Surgeon's Guide To Improve Your Life From The Inside Out gives them the ammunition for that fight.

101 Ways to Feel and Look Great! is a book for both women and men. Mothers and fathers can read it and apply the concepts not only to themselves but to their children.

People want and need some sort of personal plan to guide them now and into the future. Dr. Maximovich's 101 Ways to Feel and Look Great! fulfills that need. This guide will become your personal plan and the framework upon which you can build a better life.

Your inner thoughts, your health and how you look and feel are all related to each other. Dr. Maximovich's insights into this complex array of issues will allow you to see things in a more simple and organized way. You will be able to move forward with excitement, hope and the knowledge of how to better yourself.

101 Ways to Feel and Look Great! 3rd Edition is destined to be a primary resource for all of you who have realized, "I want to make positive changes in my life, but what can I do to make myself feel and look great?"

*****